Analytic Listening in Clinical Dialogue

Analytic Listening in Clinical Dialogue focuses on the work of four leading clinicians as they assess how their unconscious basic assumptions impact their clinical work.

Using the case study of a seven-year-old boy, the authors evaluate a videotaped psychoanalytic first interview and exchange their mutual clinical approaches. Their discussions uncover the way that unconscious basic assumptions arise from the core of one's personality and act as the pillars that support primary- and secondary-process thinking. These fundamental models of thought and emotion result in convictions which play a key role in the processes of understanding, evaluating, classifying, anticipating and regulating. The authors show how an 'analytic listening' approach can also be used to good effect in supervisions and intervisions, as it provides a path out of the domain of 'being right' into a space of what is shared as well as what is different. They argue that this method allows an analyst's own blind spots to be reduced.

Translated from the original German, *Analytic Listening in Clinical Dialogue* will be of great interest to psychoanalysts, psychotherapists and psychologists.

Dieter Bürgin is a psychoanalyst for children, adolescents and adults in private practice based in Basel, Switzerland. He is the former head of the Department for Child and Adolescent Psychiatry at the University of Basel.

Angelika Staehle is a psychoanalyst for children, adolescents and adults in private practice in Darmstadt, Germany. She is the former chair of the IPA Psychoanalytic Education Committee.

Kerstin Westhoff is a psychoanalytic psychotherapist and clinical psycho-oncologist at University Children's Hospital Basel, Switzerland.

Anna Wyler von Ballmoos is a psychoanalyst for children, adolescents and adults in private practice, based in Bern, Switzerland.

Routledge Focus on Mental Health

Routledge Focus on Mental Health presents short books on current topics, linking in with cutting-edge research and practice.

For a full list of titles in this series, please visit https://www.routledge.com/Routledge-Focus-on-Mental-Health/book-series/RFMH

Analytic Listening in Clinical Dialogue

Basic Assumptions

**Dieter Bürgin, Angelika Staehle,
Kerstin Westhoff and
Anna Wyler von Ballmoos**

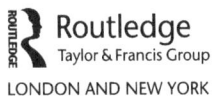

Routledge
Taylor & Francis Group

LONDON AND NEW YORK

First published in English 2023
by Routledge
4 Park Square, Milton Park, Abingdon, Oxon OX14 4RN

and by Routledge
605 Third Avenue, New York, NY 10158

Routledge is an imprint of the Taylor & Francis Group, an informa business

© 2023 Dieter Bürgin, Angelika Staehle, Kerstin Westhoff and Anna Wyler von Ballmoos

Translated by Sophie Leighton

The right of Dieter Bürgin, Angelika Staehle, Kerstin Westhoff and Anna Wyler von Ballmoos to be identified as authors of this work has been asserted in accordance with sections 77 and 78 of the Copyright, Designs and Patents Act 1988.

Published in German by Brandes & Apsel, Frankfurt, Germany, 2020

British Library Cataloguing-in-Publication Data
A catalogue record for this book is available from the British Library

Library of Congress Cataloging-in-Publication Data
A catalog record has been requested for this book

ISBN: 978-1-032-26959-7 (hbk)
ISBN: 978-1-032-30288-1 (pbk)
ISBN: 978-1-003-30434-0 (ebk)

DOI: 10.4324/9781003304340

Typeset in Times New Roman
by Deanta Global Publishing Services, Chennai, India

Contents

1 Introduction

*Happiness comes from
thinking together!*

In most analysts' experience, a report about an analytic treatment can be received in a wide variety of ways and differently realised according to the concepts applied. Depending on whether the 'material' is understood in a Kleinian, Bionian or Freudian way, or following some other school, different kinds of understanding, and accordingly various kinds of technical ways of proceeding, ensue. Why is that?

While on the one hand, the metapsychological theoretical edifice of psychoanalysis has become unified over the past hundred years, on the other hand—following its proponents' conscious and much stronger unconscious basic assumptions—it has also differentiated into many kinds of branches.

Unconscious basic assumptions arise from the core of the personality and are the pillars that support primary- and secondary-process thinking and so also the nature of all an individual's affects and phantasies. They are revealed in basic convictions, mostly not further explored, which play a key role in the processes of understanding, evaluating, classifying, anticipating and regulating. To some extent, these become consciously accessible to us in reflection or corresponding processes. We usually characterise this with phrases such as 'that's just how I see it!', 'in my view it's this or that!', 'I'm convinced that …' or 'I can't help but …'.

Some aspects of our own unconscious basic assumptions become conscious and clear to us during the process of our own analysis. Others push towards consciousness during the existential processes of their own lives and so towards subjective perception. Mostly, however, they remain, like a background programme, constantly active and comparable to Lewin's (1953) 'dream screen'; they influence all an individual's or a group's intrapsychic and interpersonal processes in a critical way and—like a well-functioning organ—scarcely become perceptible without specific consideration.

DOI: 10.4324/9781003304340-1

A sentence like the one above can be understood as the quintessence of many experiences and perceptions. But it also inevitably contains a multiplicity of basic assumptions belonging to the person writing it and, should it be read, also the person reading it.

In the groups established by Faimberg,[1] the attempt is made to explore clinical material in terms of the basic assumptions according to which each group member understands the clinical episodes presented, which hypotheses about the presenter's basic assumptions arise in each individual, which basic assumptions may be contained in the corresponding patients' statements and, finally, which basic assumptions each group member develops about the other group members' interventions and their potential basic assumptions.

In this kind of discussion, participants cannot avoid some of their self-evident, assured theoretical knowledge being put in question. They gradually reach a basic assumption that no one possesses 'the truth'; not only is it interesting to explore a counterpart's fundamental elements of thinking, feeling and wishing, but the confrontation with the other's differentness makes our own even clearer.

As a working group, this paper's four contributing authors set themselves the task over four weekend meetings of discussing each other's basic assumptions and different receptions of clinical material, using a transcribed initial video-recorded interview with a child. The process was experienced by all participants as very stimulating, as positions of 'being right' and rivalry quickly gave way to creative excitement, interest and the enjoyment of exploration. In reciprocal discourse, not only our own more or less conscious basic assumptions became clear but also, triggered by the group members' questions to each other, our own, hitherto unconscious, basic assumptions also came to light.

In the first round, the problem of basic assumptions was discussed. Afterwards the video was watched several times in short episodes. Every episode, as well as the sequence of the episodes, was discussed intensively, with great enjoyment as well as appropriate seriousness. Each participant composed a first draft of his own way of understanding and experiences while reflecting on his own basic assumptions. The group discussed these reports in depth using the interview transcript and only then received the basic amnestic data. The group therefore had not only a shared text available but also the commonly experienced images in the video scenes. This initially eased the exchange, but as it progressed they all used the text and images more than the video as a basis. Finally, it was decided that the key points of the experiences should be summarised in a publication. This way of proceeding may serve to stimulate interested readers to pursue the processes in a group as well, to form their own picture and gain more clarity for themselves about their own basic assumptions. In supervisions and intervisions, this procedure can certainly also be used to good effect, as it provides a path out of the domain of 'being right' into a space of what is shared as well as what is different, allows our own blind spots—at least partly—to be removed and increases the appeal of considering the same phenomenon from various perspectives.

References

Faimberg H. (2019): Basic theoretical assumptions underpinning 'Faimberg's method 'Listening to listening'. *Int. J. Psychoanalysis*, 100/3, 447–426.

Lewin B. D. (1953): Reconsideration of the dream screen. *Psychoanal. Quarterly*, 22/2, 179–199.

Note

1 Faimberg's method (2019): listening to listening.

2   Basic assumptions

The *psyche* cannot be objectivised in any satisfactory way. *Psychologism* corresponds to the need to be still able to objectivise it comprehensively. It considers the models of understanding used to be the exemplary truth of reality and therefore tolerates nothing else alongside it. But neither mythology, religion nor philosophy constitute a *scientific psychology*. *Cultural development* can be understood as a process that begins with mythological concepts and ends in a streamlined science. 'Because the life of the mind—however that is understood—can never be satisfactorily objectivised, debate arises concerning the objectivising concepts and methods' (Saner, 1999, p. 197).

A self is presented in a highly differentiated way; 'reality is not guaranteed primarily by the "common nature" of all men who constitute it' (Arendt, 2018, p. 57). 'Being seen and being heard by others derive their significance from the fact that everybody sees and hears from a different position' (p. 57). The reality of the public sphere arises from 'the simultaneous presence of innumerable perspectives and aspects in which the common world presents itself and for which no common measurement or denominator can ever be devised' (p. 57). 'The end of the common world has come when it is seen only under one aspect and is permitted to present itself in only one perspective' (p. 58).

The formation of basic assumptions corresponds to a fundamental, proto-mental activity that may even be prenatally constituted. Basic assumptions develop from extremely early scenarios characterised by relationships to partial objects, primary symbolisations, psychotic anxieties and splitting mechanisms, as well as projective identification. Basic assumptions have their own distinct goals, such as the striving for dependence/independence, fight or flight, or formation of a couple. They are not orientated by knowledge or even science but by primary thinking activities. In proto-mental systems, there may be prototypes of the three basic assumptions that can often be found in groups. A lack of structure in a group allows basic assumptions to push forward.

DOI: 10.4324/9781003304340-2

As a form of sub-system of the ego (Gill and Brenman, 1966), the individual, a biologically constituted gregarious animal, so with strong social relatedness, forms a proto-mentality at a very early stage that extends to groups but later loses its power through subsequent intellectual endeavours. There is probably an interplay here between biologically constituted and socially acquired factors. Basic assumptions have a survival value for the individual and the group. As irrational, fundamental convictions, basic assumptions interconnect the members of every group in an unconscious way (Bürgin, 2017). In such groups, any kind of development process is lacking, 'For basic assumptions become dangerous in proportion as the attempt is made to translate them into action' (Bion, 1961, p. 157). Participation in action according to a basic assumption occurs spontaneously and intuitively.

Psychoanalytic conceptualising, theorising and thinking are also based on more or less explicit basic assumptions. In connection with group phenomena, Bion in particular has made reference to this fact. At the various developmental stages of thinking, imagining and fantasising, the attempt is made to apply assumptions that have once proved favourable to new experiences as well. Primary- and secondary-process procedures therefore make different contributions to this. Most of these basic assumptions are subject to *primary infantile amnesia* but still remain fully available to the ego's emotional-cognitive activities as aids to classifying and understanding. *Careful reflection* and *creative exchange* about basic assumptions present in analysts are not highly popular. For they are unsettling, require putting things in question and presuppose tolerance. As they can never be satisfactorily objectivised, they seem to prejudice the development of theory and the evaluation of affiliations. The alternative, though, is an ungracious battle between 'dukes, princes, kings and emperors' that is not conducive to scientific thinking in psychoanalysis. So basic assumptions exist in a more or less conscious way not only in relation to *theory* and the *genesis of disorders* but also in relation to the *psychoanalytic situation*, or *attitude, as well as the psychoanalytic process* itself.

In his considerations of group activities, Bion worked from the premise of three *fixed, diametrically opposed and fundamental basic assumptions* (fight/flight; dependence/independence; singularity/pair formation) that instigate the development of adversely functioning groups that are not actually able to work and are clearly distinguishable from 'working groups' that follow no such rigid model.

Our group clearly understood the concept of basic assumptions more widely and openly, namely as a sum of fundamental, explicit and implicit 'views', convictions, representations and attitudes, permeated by many kinds of emotions that continually accompany our psychoanalytic working and accompany us constantly as more or less integrated theories and 'insights'. Without special effort, though, they are not communicated, although they extensively influence our conceptualising and intervening.

The curious, good-willed exchange about this and a tactful exploration in this domain proved to be exciting and enjoyable. This may be connected with the fact that the group members were sympathetically attached to each other and liked working together. How far the constellation of three women and one man contributed something further to that dynamic cannot, without comparison, be precisely assessed.

2.1 Basic assumptions and the individual

Most polar basic assumptions, such as that the subject either functions as a passive receptacle that is filled with external world or it manifests itself as an independent unity with its own autonomous metabolism, should not be seen in terms of *either/or* but *both/and*.

Our *psychoanalytic procedure* is guided by our *implicit and explicit basic assumptions*. So the question constantly arises as to the level of functioning at which communicative elements originating from the analysand are 'heard' and taken up by the analyst in accordance with his own basic assumptions.

As concerns the analytic processes, we all have *implicit basic assumptions*. Psychoanalytic circles have been—and unfortunately often still are now—concerned with *struggles for supremacy of one or other of the basic assumptions*. For decades, attempts have also been made to explain the unconscious basic assumptions that accompany us either in *low-frequency or high-frequency psychoanalytic proceedings*.

2.2 Basic assumptions and questions of treatment technique

Also in relation to treatment technique in the clinical domain, we are guided by our basic assumptions: for example, that there is a need to *create a protected intermediate space* that allows for playing and the use of an object, exercising the capacity to be alone in another's presence in a related way and new formations of old relational constellations in the transference. Here the analyst's interpretation of the patient's intrapsychic events is much less prominent than his subjective perception and reflection (in the sense of self-critical reflection) on the *current self-experience in this specific situation*. Our own thoughts and sensations as that which are manifestly present, partly shaped by past events, allow the *experience of relatedness and separateness at the same time*, as well as new levels of freedom in *closeness and distance*.

If, for example, a patient *brings no capacity to open a virtual interme-diate space*, the *construction of a virtual intermediate space* may be the first step in the process. If a virtual intermediate space is *obliterated* by the patient's pathology (e.g. compulsive filling of the virtual intermediate space that allows the counterpart no room at all, or by the opposite, or by distor-tions), dismantling the obliteration and *establishing the capacity to play* are a primary goal. If there is a *usable virtual intermediate space*, the principal goal consists of *letting a more or less creative play arise*, in which *from two separately functioning but related individuals a repeatedly new, commonly shared third emerges*, which can be symbolised and constantly opens up new pathways.

What are *the only partly conscious 'basic assumptions'* that lie at the basis of our conceptualising? What does the corresponding *conception of man* that we bring into the process, like it or not, resemble? What considera-tion should be given to our *conscious and unconscious way of listening to our patients*? For our 'listening' determines our speaking!

Our technique of listening, understanding and transforming what is reported to us by the patient cannot be thought about independently of a the-ory or basic assumptions, whether these are implicit or explicit. Of course, anyone engaged in clinical work has to record, always very painfully, that in the deepening of the process not nearly as much depends on which tech-nique we use as on whether we manage to perceive the non-conscious trends in the transference—which of course is another basic assumption!

The setting begins to speak when it is reflected on. It reflects our *basic assumptions about symbolisation*, even if it is about the *playing* that serves as a *vehicle of the transference* and where *symbolisation, above all the pri-mary kind*, is frequently shown at the *motoric level*. The setting allows the transmission of *archaic messages about the body* (facial expressions, atti-tude, way of moving, tonus etc.) as well as about *actions* (rhythm, speed). More complex, more developed 'communications' find expression through *thing- and word-representations and narrative scenic envelopes* in the transference—in the *asymmetrical presence of an other*.

Even during reflection on the *relations between body and psyche*, i.e. also on the *corresponding disturbances*, the conscious or unconscious *basic assumptions of those reflecting* play a major role. For these basic assump-tions form something like *axioms*, on *the foundation of which correspond-ing theories* are constructed. Although the body functions according to primarily *biological laws* with their vast complexity, and the *psyche evinces different structuring and ordering principles*, it is one of our basic assump-tions that *there is no psychic process that is divorced from biology, but that the psyche also receives infinitely much information from the body, only a small part of which reaches consciousness.*

If there is *no exchange with the counterpart about each individual's unavoidable basic assumptions, co-creativity* dries up. This conveys *another perspective* and *other vertices*, allowing the *emergence of new basic assumptions* and supporting *self-reflection*.

2.3 Basic assumptions and social orders

Natural orders are relatively stable, whereas man-made orders are not. These are based on commonly shared mythologies and in constant danger of collapse. They are often maintained over a long period, sometimes with violence, terror and force, as long as enough people believe in the corresponding basic assumptions and base-ideologies. If it is as it were created by the gods, it appears indestructible.

Myths and basic assumptions, for example about gods and human beings, rulers and subjects or a classification of human beings (into e.g. free, unfree or slaves), formed a kind of cement for such basic structures. From this, social norms and laws could be developed as the foundations of law (e.g. the codex of King Hammurabi in Assyria in 1700 BC), which promised, with corresponding obedience and observance of the rules, that a safe and peaceful as well as just life would be possible.

Every world-historical view is based on the infinitely diverse configurations and manifold powerful developments of often rather unclearly expressed basic assumptions and the resulting world views of larger or smaller collectives. The attempt to combine psychoanalytic thinking and conceptualising and an associated set of basic assumptions with contemporary world-political questions (as undertaken by e.g. Sklar in his book published in 2019) also contains an embryonic attempt to apply the elucidation, application and discussion of basic assumptions concerning forms of human relationships to current world events. As this set of themes is not in the foreground here however, it will not be further explored at this point, although such an undertaking would certainly have some attractions.

2.4 Basic assumptions and the group

The individual has a tendency and a capacity to connect *involuntarily and quickly with other individuals*, which indicates the existence of a protomental system. When a group has gathered together under certain basic assumptions, it has—like a family—become *something real that is part of human life*. But it is not at all the same as a family.

Basic assumptions exclude everything else and *do not seek to adopt any other standpoints* or even understand them. They are based not on knowledge or even science, but on magical thinking. Independent thinking is denigrated as rebellion and stifled at birth.

According to Bion, there is a distinction to be drawn between basic-assumption groups and work groups. It is only in work groups that a co-created cooperative context prevails.

Strong fundamental affects form a cement that binds together basic-assumption groups (e.g. guilt and depression, hope of rescue, rage and hatred). People with similar basic assumptions come together effortlessly and spontaneously. Groupings of this kind cause a group to be quickly structured in the way that suits it to act according to the predominant basic assumptions. There is a fierce resistance to any learning from experience, even a hatred of any developmental process. Basic-assumption groups offer the illusion of allowing individual identity to merge into the collective. The immersion in the group is supposed to convey security and revitalisation as well as an inalterable belonging.

A truly 'differentiated group' is synonymous with a 'work group'. Work groups are formed to carry out specific tasks. They establish procedural rules for this. Its members are convinced of the value of relational or scientific data. Verbal exchange and the special use of communicative symbols are typical of work groups. The less a group corresponds to a work group, i.e. the more it becomes a basic-assumption group, the less it makes rational use of verbal communication and mainly uses the mode of action. Work groups are willing to learn from experience.

Development is therefore a key characteristic that distinguishes a work group from a basic-assumption group. But its endeavours to carry out an immediate task are constantly hindered by affective drive forces of obscure origin. Work groups can therefore also be hampered by powerful emotional strivings. Basic-assumption groups and work groups are poles on a continuum with many intermediate points. Nevertheless, a consideration of the poles makes it easier to reflect on what is happening in a group.

As soon as the individual thinks or behaves in a way that contradicts the group's basic assumptions, he experiences this as an *unpleasant effect*. So there is a '*conflict between group mentality and the desires of the individual*' (Bion, 1961, p. 60).

A basic-assumption group seems to know only two methods of self-preservation: *fight or flight*. The preservation of the species by procreation is perceived as just as important for the preservation of the group as methods of self-preservation (i.e. both are responded to with fight and/or flight). With flight, the group takes precedence, while the individual is left in the lurch if necessary. In a fight/flight group, the form of *leadership* recognised as appropriate is the one that mobilises the group *to attack someone or accompanies it in escaping*.

In *'dependent' groups, the immature individual believes he is finding security in the group.* All his worries are shifted onto the leader. Ambitious or narcissistic people create quite a lot of problems in dependent groups, though, because they begin to compete with the leader.

Working on latent basic assumptions prevents these from restricting a work group's functions. Groups that work from specific *unconscious basic assumptions* are characterised by *functional modes of the proto-mental apparatus* and so by a *primary-process form of thinking.*

References

Arendt H. (2018): *The Human Condition.* Chicago/London: University of Chicago Press.

Bion W. R. (1961): *Experiences in Groups and Other Papers.* London: Tavistock.

Bürgin D. (2017): Zur Ko-Kreation eines kooperativen Kontextes [On the co-creation of a cooperative context]. In: Harms A./Hartmann H.P. (eds.): *Einsamkeit. Jahrb. d. Selbstpsychologie.* Frankfurt: Brandes & Apsel, pp. 178–190.

Gill, M. M. and Brenman M. (1966): *Hypnosis and Related States. Psychoanalytic Studies in Regression.* New York: Wiley.

Saner H. (1999): Die Nebel [The mists]. In: *Macht und Ohnmacht der Symbole.* Basel: Lenos.

Sklar J. (2019): *Dark Times. Psychoanalytic Perspectives on Politics, History and Mourning.* London: Phoenix.

3 The interview (Simone, aged seven years and seven months)

This is the verbatim transcript of a video-recording made in front of a one-way mirror. For the purpose of our discussions, it was selected from a large number of conversations, less for an intrinsic event or content that makes it distinctive than to have an easily comprehensible, common and reproducible basis for our conversations with a child in the 'latency' period.

The conversation with the boy hospitalised in a child psychiatry and psychotherapy department was presented by the first author for diagnostic reasons. Behind the one-way mirror sat a group of specialists, some of whom were known to Simone, with whom the diagnostic evaluation was discussed afterwards. The layout of the place was familiar to Simone. He had been given detailed information verbally before the conversation, and his agreement was sought for the setting as a whole. Simone agreed that a group of people could participate in the conversation behind the one-way mirror, and he was informed that this conversation was a one-time event. It was therefore a matter of allowing a meaningful encounter to take place while also making the best possible use of the limited nature of the contact.

To guarantee confidentiality, all personal data (in particular concerning his environment) have been anonymised as far as possible. So we will call the patient Simon.

Simone: Why can't we hear those people over there?
Interviewer: That's how it's been arranged. But we don't have to pay any attention to them.
(Some information follows about the one-way mirror and a small adjoining room that people can enter and look out from.)
Simone: But people are well hidden there. I'd be happy if I were in there *(in the room behind the one-way mirror)*.
Interviewer: And who would you look at then?
Simone: You.

DOI: 10.4324/9781003304340-3

Interviewer: Me? Aha!

Simone: Or someone else.

Interviewer: Really? And what would you want to know if you looked?

Simone: Don't know!

Interviewer: Are you a good observer?

Simone: Mm ... Yes!

Interviewer: Yes? Have you got used to observing people? And would you actually like to be there, but so that you can't be seen? Like under a magic cloak?

Simone: Mm.

Interviewer: And are people not to see you because they shouldn't know you want to know something?

Simone: (nods) Why don't we do it the other way round: they can sit here, and we'll sit over there?

Interviewer: Yes, well, you know, that's just the way it's been arranged for us now. But I see you'd like it to be the other way round, so we'd observe these people or you could observe me ...

Simone: Yes!

Interviewer: ... Perhaps we can come back a bit now ... what we're doing now is easy after all, in fact so we can get to know each other a little ...

(Simone gets up and examines a small side room with a small one-way mirror.)

Simone: Hold on, now I can't see the mirror there ... not at all.

Interviewer: Yes, not at all, it's dark there. Come, please sit down again.

Simone: I can see through a bit there.

Interviewer: Just a very little, yes.

Simone: It's black there ...

Interviewer: So, the aim of what the two of us are doing now is to get to know each other a bit. And so I'm happy if you ...

Simone: Could we draw something?

Interviewer: Mm ... if you'd like to show something of yourself to me ...

Simone: Yes.

Interviewer: Would you perhaps like to tell me first why you've actually come to us?

Simone: Er ... I did something stupid!

Interviewer: Because you did something stupid? Can you tell me a bit more about it? What is 'doing something stupid'?

Simone: Mm ... isn't it just that you want to confuse me a bit, so that I say more?

Interviewer: I'm happy for you to tell me more, but I don't want to confuse you.

Simone: Yes you do.

Interviewer: I do?

Simone: Yes!

Interviewer: No, there you're doing something to me, you know, just like that ...

Simone: But you would!

Interviewer: ... and you don't believe what I'm telling you at all.

Simone: No, not at all!

Interviewer: Then we already have a problem together, you see. Because you're saying I'm just as you think I am. That means you're not at all bothered about what I'm really like. Why should I want to confuse you then?

Simone: Simple ...

Interviewer: What would that mean for me?

Simone: Don't know either.

Interviewer: But, you know, perhaps there's something in you that sometimes confuses you?

Simone: Mm ...

Interviewer: Can you concentrate well?

Simone: Yes.

Interviewer: Yes? You can stay with one thing?

Simone: (nods)

Interviewer: Yes? There's nothing in you that confuses you?

Simone: Yes, there is.

Interviewer: What?

Simone: When people keep not answering me.

Interviewer: I don't completely understand. When someone doesn't give you an answer or when someone keeps giving you an answer ...?

Simone: (nods)

Interviewer: You shouldn't be given an answer?

Simone: (nods)

Interviewer: Now I don't understand at all anymore.

Simone: Tee-hee!

Interviewer: So, we've already got to know something else, which is, if you make sure the other person ...

Simone: ... let's draw, let's draw!!

Interviewer: ... if you make sure the other person is not coming out any more, then you can stay under a magic cloak. But that could mean you're actually very afraid someone might discover you.

Simone: Hm ... *(indicating no).*

Interviewer: If you stay under the magic cloak, then no one can know who Simone is.

Simone: Yes, they can.

Interviewer: Are people allowed to know that?

Simone: Yes.

Interviewer: Because there's a strong wish after all for someone to know who Simone is?

Simone: To know who <u>you</u> are!

Interviewer: Okay, you may know that too, so let's get to know each other a little, shall we? Perhaps we'll do that now just with a drawing.

Simone: Mm …

Interviewer: Good. Shall we play a drawing game?[1] I'll make a squiggle, and you look and see what you'd like to develop from it. Then you make a squiggle, and I'll look to see what I can make from it. Now you just have to tell me who should do the first squiggle.

Simone: Er, you!

Interviewer: I? Good *(Interviewer makes a squiggle).* Now you can make whatever you want from it!

Simone: I don't understand what I could do.

Interviewer: You can make something out of this squiggle, exactly what you'd like at the moment. You can complete it by drawing anything you want.

Simone: (draws) So now it's your turn.

Interviewer: Yes, what have you just made?

Simone: Don't know either.

Interviewer: You know, you could make something you already know, so you'd know what it is …

Simone: Okay, but something much better than a squiggle …

Interviewer: Yes, we'll just have to see … then make something else. I'd just started with that … You could try out a squiggle …

Simone: (draws for a bit longer)

Interviewer: So, when you say something better than a squiggle … did you have the feeling that my squiggle isn't right, isn't good for you?

Simone: I don't understand what you mean *(shaking his head).*

Interviewer: Aha, so you know I don't mean anything at all yet, but the squiggle is just something you can create something from. Now you've made a car! A car with a light at the front and an antenna on top.

Simone: Mm, that's an antenna where there's a mophead on it.

Interviewer: What do you mean by that, a mophead? A mophead-antenna like that?

Simone: Yes.

Interviewer: Mm, would you like to tell me a bit about your car?

Simone: Something else can be drawn on here too, here at the front.
Interviewer: Mm ...?
Simone: A horn.
Interviewer: Aha.
Simone: Or a car-megaphone.
Interviewer: Yes?
Simone: (draws)
Interviewer: So there's a lorry in front with 'KABEA' written on it.
Simone: KPA!
Interviewer: KPA, ah! ... that stands for the children's psychiatry department,[2] so that means it has something to do with our department?
Simone: Mm.
Interviewer: And the car's hooting because it wants to get past?
Simone: Wait a moment *(he draws)*, I must draw something next to it that's different from what it is now ...
Interviewer: What would you like now? Also to write KPA?
Simone: No, I must write something other than KPA there—ambulance!
Interviewer: Aha! Mm.
Simone: That's better than KPA!
Interviewer: So actually that's an ambulance that wants to drive on and the other one is getting in the way a bit ...
Simone: ... wait, there's something else!
Interviewer: Mm, who's in the ambulance then?
Simone: An emergency man.
Interviewer: An emergency man. Has something happened?
Simone: Yes.
Interviewer: What then?
Simone: An accident!
Interviewer: An accident?
Simone: On the motorway.
Interviewer: What kind of accident was it?
Simone: A car accident.
Interviewer: Ah.
Simone: A crash.
Interviewer: And ...
Simone: He's switched on the sirens—now you make something!
Interviewer: I'd just like to understand that properly first, because actually ... you're saying it has to do with the KPA. So that's an ambulance and it has something to do with the KPA?

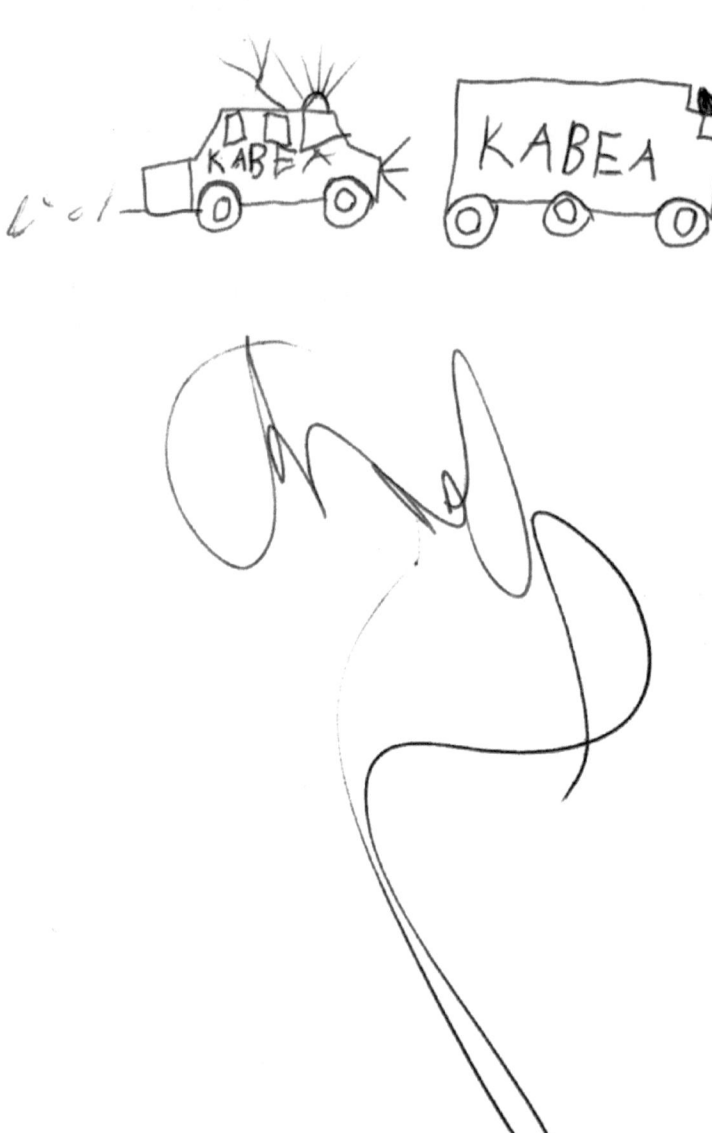

Squiggle 1.

Simone: Yes.

Interviewer: So, actually there's been an accident with a child there?

Simone: One from the KPA!

Interviewer: From the KPA?

Simone: Yes!

Interviewer: And help is urgently needed.

Simone: Yes.

Interviewer: Do you think it could be that Simone is actually telling me he may urgently need help?

Simone: Urgently? *(shakes his head)*

Interviewer: Not so urgently? But all the same?

Simone: I think so!

Interviewer: Good, that's an important story you're telling me!

Simone: Can I also make a street?

Interviewer: Yes, but wait, now it's my turn, no, now it's your turn to make a squiggle ... Then I'll look to see what I can make of this one, shall I? Shall we have a small exhibition?

Simone: Hm?

Interviewer: Down here *(on the ground)*, where we can easily see ourselves. Now you could make the squiggle, and I can look there to see what I could make from this one.

Simone: (draws) A big squiggle!

Interviewer: That's a big squiggle, right, yes!

Simone: And I already know what it is.

Interviewer: You know what it is? Well then you can just complete the squiggle yourself if you like.

Simone: Some water!

Interviewer: Hm?

Simone: Water.

Interviewer: Water that's doing something?

Simone: ... that's going upwards.

Interviewer: Waves, do you think?

Simone: Yes.

Interviewer: Aha, waves of water!

Simone: Wait, I could put something in there *(draws)*—I'll draw the scales.

Interviewer: Mm, so the little fish is swimming in these high waves?

Simone: Mm!

Interviewer: Mm.

Simone: Oh, you must also see the fish's mother, it's big *(draws)*, oops, down there I'm making a big fish *(draws)*.

Interviewer: So actually they're both in a stormy sea now.

Simone: Mm.

Interviewer: Where it goes up high. And how do they cope with the storm?

Simone: Cope with it?

Interviewer: Yes.

Simone: Because at the front it's slowly getting less critical now, look.

Interviewer: Ah, it's quietening down there?

Simone: Yes.

Interviewer: Mm.

Simone: Do you know how it comes so quickly?

Interviewer: No.

Simone: Does that come so quickly?

Interviewer: I don't know.

Simone: From the hurricane!

Interviewer: Yes?

Simone: Inside.

Interviewer: The hurricane has made the high waves.

Simone: Aha.

Interviewer: And then it's ... ah ... do you think we could say Simone had perhaps gone through some very stormy times with his Mummy?

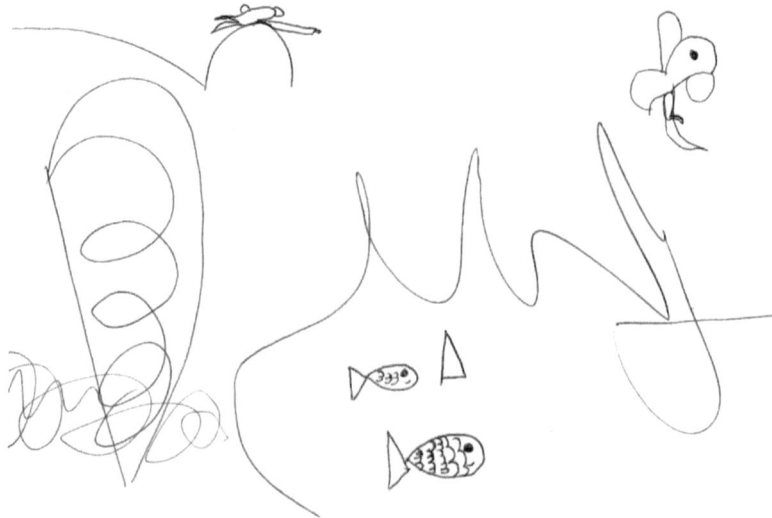

Squiggle 2.

Simone: Hm ... *(shaking his head).*

Interviewer: That can't be said?

Simone: No.

Interviewer: Is that wrong, do you think?

Simone: (nods) Ah. Well yes, yes actually.

Interviewer: That's right after all, is it?

Simone: Ah, what else could we make ...

Interviewer: Then that was a difficult time you've both had ...

Simone: ... and I can also *(draws, breathes loudly, draws some more)* ... do you know, do you know about those things that *(touches his neck)* have a bag on there?

Interviewer: Yes, the pelican!

Simone: Yes, a pelican, but I can't draw it any better.

Interviewer: Yes—but that's good!

Simone: Now you can draw something! *(pushes the drawing-pad over to the interviewer)*

Interviewer: Can you tell me anything else about the pelican? What's it doing there now?

Simone: It wants to catch the fish.

Interviewer: Oh, now the storm is certainly behind them, but where it seems to be quietening down ...

Simone: Yes?

Interviewer: ... there's a danger, and the pelican may snap up one or both of them.

Simone: Yes, now something dangerous is coming with the pelican.

Interviewer: Ah, yes?

Simone: Yes!

Interviewer: What is it?

Simone: A hill, this is a man, he's carrying ... a gun because he's protecting the fish.

Interviewer: Aha, and there he could shoot at the pelican now?

Simone: Yes!

Interviewer: So, first it was very dangerous for you and now it becomes very dangerous for him.

Simone: Mm.

Interviewer: Aha.

Simone: But there could be something else.

Interviewer: What?

Simone: What else could be made? Ah yes. There's a wall, then you put your head in there.

Interviewer: Mm?

Simone: ... and they can get to the other side of the sea; the fish don't have to experience the threatening danger; they can get through there. But they have to go a long way down ... and then a long way up, as far as they have to go down.

Interviewer: ... as they have to go down.

Simone: And there, as they have to go up.

Interviewer: ... where they have to go up.

Simone: Up to there.

Interviewer: Aha, and then are they rescued there?

Simone: Yes, in the other sea above.

Interviewer: Aha!

Simone: Could we make another story now?

Interviewer: Yes of course ... but that's a great story you've told me there, a very important one. I think that's a very exciting story you've made there, Simone, really!

Simone: How many stories could be made?

Interviewer: Well, actually as many as we have time for, we still have a good half hour left.

Simone: Why not longer?

Interviewer: Well, because, then our time is up.

Simone: What could we make? You draw something, another pelican or something, or a little fish.

Interviewer: Do you think I should also draw a little fish or a pelican? Ah, then I'll make something else? *(Interviewer draws).*

Simone: Ah, a fox!

Interviewer: Ah, you've already seen that? You saw this shape quickly. Incredible how quick you are, how quickly you've recognised the shape! What do you think about it?

Simone: Hmm, the mark could also be put underneath it ... and there we could also ... could you just give me the blue pencil a moment? *(i.e. the interviewer's pencil).*

Interviewer: Mm ... just a moment!

Simone: (draws) ... a small, a big opening like that ... I only want, now do you see what's there?

Interviewer: I'm excited to see!

Simone: That's the fox's den.

Interviewer: So it is!

Simone: And he can't get through it any more ... because there's some treasure he wants to dig out with a spade, look now—we have a spade.

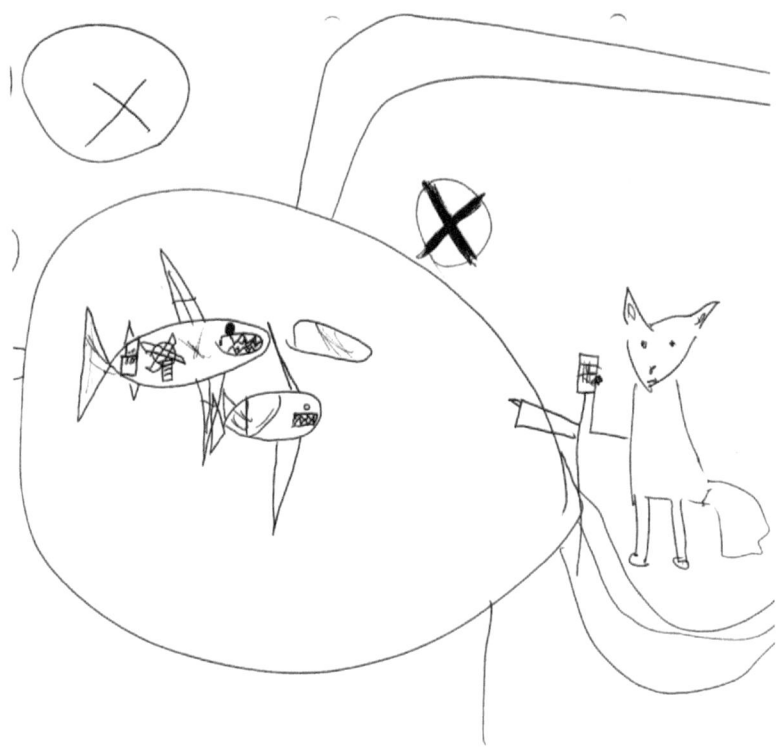

Squiggle 3.

Interviewer: Mm.
Simone: And just look a moment, he wants to do this in the night.
Interviewer: Aha!
Simone: And then I'll make a little mouth …
Interviewer: Ah …
Simone: So, and there's the fox's mouth.
Interviewer: Aha.
Simone: There are the eyes.
Interviewer: Mm.
Simone: There's the mouth.
Interviewer: Mm.
Simone: Now it's getting a bit dangerous for the fox!
Interviewer: Aha … why's that?
Simone: Or a bit for the fish, with sharp teeth, bigger, so many.

Interviewer: Mm.

Simone: How can we draw a shark?

Interviewer: You've drawn it there, that's already a shark, just as you've drawn it's good.

Simone: But how can a shark be made from that?

Interviewer: Yes, you know, they're also long and thin like that, and then they have a big fin on their backs.

Simone: Do you think ...?

Interviewer: Yes, like that, that's great.

Simone: And then there.

Interviewer: And then a triangle, for a fin on its back ... mm.

Simone: And then it has another pair at the back there.

Interviewer: Yes, it has small fins at the back too ... mm.

Simone: and then ... how can we, er, do the mouth?

Interviewer: I think it's a good mouth that you've drawn there; I'd make a similar one for the shark, that goes perhaps back to there, you know.

Simone: To there?

Interviewer: Mm.

Simone: They have double teeth.

Interviewer: Mm, a double row.

Simone: Why a double row?

Interviewer: So when the front ones break off, they still have a row left. They have a whole lot of rows of teeth, not just a double one, they have up to ten rows!

Simone: They're lucky, they have more than we do, because we only have one set of teeth!

Interviewer: Yes, but twice; you're getting some new teeth through now aren't you? You've already had some teeth fall out and now you have some new ones!

Simone: No, oh yes, one at the back, and there are two more there.

Interviewer: Yes, but you already have lots of new ones.

Simone: Mm ... more there, a bit, then a bit there, and we'll put a bit in the middle ... that's a skull on him.

Interviewer: Aha, has he drawn it on or is that one he's half-eaten?

Simone: One he's eaten, a bit, or it's still alive.

Interviewer: It's still alive?

Simone: Yes, a person has got it out and put a plaster on it, look, it must be a huge plaster *(draws)*. There, in the middle, a few dots, that's its plaster.

Interviewer: The skull is still alive, is it?

Simone: No, I've, it's drawn something on it.

Interviewer: Ah, it's been drawn on, and does the shark have a plaster there?

Simone: Yes, because someone's hurt it.

Interviewer: Aha.

Simone: That's its child, it already has a few little fins on its back, but they're already long, look.

Interviewer: Aha.

Simone: It already has long fins on its back, the child.

Interviewer: Yes, it's already become a proper shark then; these two harmless little fish ...

Simone: Mm.

Interviewer: ... have suddenly become two little predator fish!

Simone: No—or yes!

Interviewer: Yes.

Simone: We must double it with that one, look now. But then they'll swim up to the head if they want to get in.

Interviewer: Ah, that's it there, aha.

Simone: Then we could make it better: on the way they ate a lot, then they became little predator fish. Look now, that's the way—then they became proper little predator fish. At first they were really pretty, they were happy, and now they're really big—and, aha, there's the fox with the door. Let's make another story!

Interviewer: Yes, there's another thing I'd just like to understand quickly— did the fox actually want to get the treasure but couldn't get across?

Simone: Yes.

Interviewer: Why can't he get across?

Simone: Er, because there's also a bit of water there.

Interviewer: Aha, and he can't get through there.

Simone: Yes, and there too.

Interviewer: And there too?

Simone: That's the boundary they've agreed and when people go across there and dig out the treasure from them, he passes out.

Interviewer: So the fox actually knows where something valuable is, but he can't get it.

Simone: Hm *(indicating no)*.

Interviewer: He can't.

Simone: Yes, but then he has a better idea.

Interviewer: Yes.

Simone: Where's the blue pencil?

Interviewer: Here!

Simone: Give it to me for a moment!

Interviewer: Does it continue there, or does it go on to a new page?

Simone: A new one will do. Then he's holding a blue gun, he's also shooting with it, look now.

Interviewer: Aha!

Simone: That's really close to them, the bullets, look!

Interviewer: Ooh—now he's shooting at the sharks.

Simone: Yes, but at first they didn't harm him at all, look.

Interviewer: Yes, so …

Simone: You know, that's the fox's mate there, that's the other side of the mountain, and now he's dug a huge hole there for the pelican so he can get through, and there the pelican has made just as big a hole, look!

Interviewer: Yes, aha.

Simone: Only he must take something else out; that's the little bridge there, then he's finished and can get through.

Interviewer: Then the pelican can get through and he gets out there.

Simone: Yes.

Interviewer: Then the pelican is near the treasure but the fox isn't.

Simone: But the fox is there too because he's shooting at them.

Interviewer: Aha, then he can get through, ah I see!

Simone: And now he has also buried some valuable treasure, do you know what?

Interviewer: No?

Simone: The sharks.

Interviewer: Ah …?

Simone: Or: better story, to conclude it. That's a stone now, isn't it?

Interviewer: Yes.

Simone: And there the fox has arranged that I dig out this treasure and you dig out mine.

Interviewer: Has he arranged that with the pelican or with someone else?

Simone: No, with the fish.

Interviewer: With the sharks?

Simone: Yes.

Interviewer: So, the sharks and the fox may get the treasure.

Simone: Yes, and then they've built another den, the fox now has the den inside there, and they now have the den inside there, they've put water in there so they can swim through, look now, now it's finished!

Interviewer: Yes, the sharks are constantly threatened and yet they still keep managing to get away.

Simone: Yes.

Interviewer: They can keep escaping …

Simone: And afterwards, in the new story, it gets really funny.

Interviewer: Good, then we'll put this drawing down here.

Simone: And now the story gets very funny.

Interviewer: Lovely, I'm excited, so, how does it look?

Simone: So, there's the great big sea again, look now, another stone like that, do you see it now?

Interviewer: Well yes, I've seen the big sea and then there's a fish, I can see that too.

Simone: And they've been made smaller, look, now the smaller one *(points to a drawn picture)* has grown up and now it's had a little baby; do you know why?

Interviewer: No.

Simone: Because the mother has died, and that was the girl.

Interviewer: Aha.

Simone: Look, it has a very small fish.

Interviewer: Aha.

Simone: Can I take this drawing away with me?

Interviewer: I wouldn't want that, but we can make a photocopy, then you can take the photocopy away.

Simone: But a blue one like that, where it looks right, grey isn't as pretty.

Interviewer: Yes, unfortunately we can't do that, the photocopier makes it black.

Simone: Ah!

Interviewer: So here some time has passed on the land, the Mummy has died, and the little girl has become a big woman, that's now just a boy, but how did this baby come about?

Simone: Those are now swordfish.

Interviewer: What?

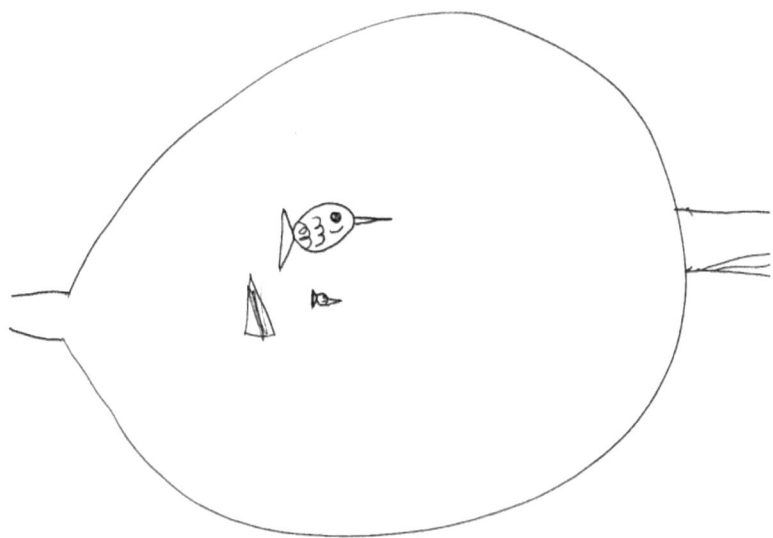

Squiggle 4.

Simone: They're swordfish.

Interviewer: Swordfish, ah right—and they can make a whole row of babies, how does that happen?

Simone: Yes?

Interviewer: Yes?

Simone: Do you know this fish?

Interviewer: That's another shark, isn't it?

Simone: Yes, just a different kind.

Interviewer: Aha!

Simone: Do you know this kind?

Interviewer: Yes, I've seen it before, those are hammerhead sharks.

Simone: Hammerhead …?

Interviewer: Hammerhead sharks.

Simone: Are they valuable?

Interviewer: I don't know, but in any case they're big and dangerous fish.

Simone: Dangerous how?

Interviewer: All sharks, you know, like to eat.

Simone: Blood!

Interviewer: And if they taste blood then especially, yes.

Simone: And he also has the baby now, just a rather smaller one than before, and he already has that kind of mouth, and then it goes on, where we can go on …

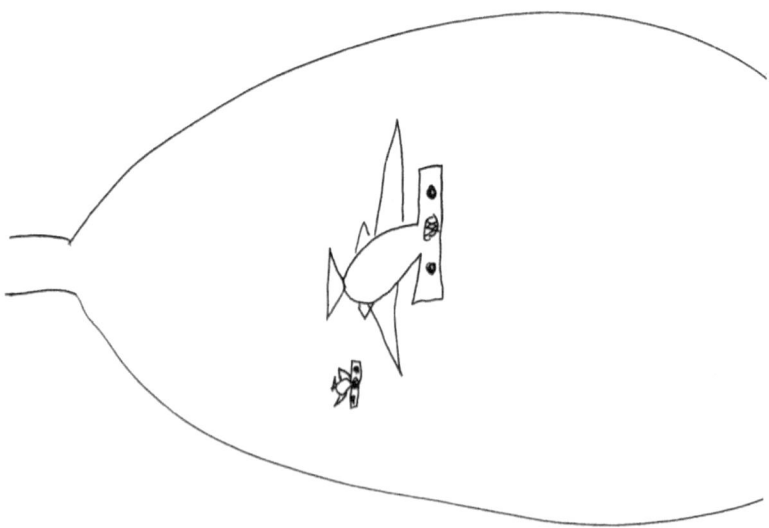

Squiggle 5.

Interviewer: What is happening with these two hammerhead sharks?

Simone: They keep turning into another fish, then another, and another, always another.

Interviewer: Aha.

Simone: In some time they will be the same again.

Interviewer: When we said before: how is it then with Simone—can he also change form and ...?

Simone: Yes, become nicer.

Interviewer: Nicer—are you bad then?

Simone: Have been!

Interviewer: Yes?

Simone: But now I realise I'm not to do it anymore. Could we play something else now?

Interviewer: Of course, but first can you tell me what's the bad thing you did, Simone?

Simone: I don't even know any more.

Interviewer: Ah, right!

Simone: These *(i.e. all the pages with squiggles)* must be collected together then.

Interviewer: Yes.

Simone: The pages ... and that's the fifth story.

Interviewer: Yes.

Simone: The fifth.

Interviewer: Yes.

Simone: Eh, does a five go like that on the page?

Interviewer: That's not quite right; a normal five, seen from your viewpoint, would be like that, can you see that?

Simone: Mm.

Interviewer: That's now been reversed in the mirror, do you see? Yes, that's the right one.

Simone: Okay, now let's play a game.

Interviewer: We only have five minutes left, so not long now. I would actually still be interested in what you did in order not to be bad anymore.

Simone: Developed further!

Interviewer: Oh, developed further! Do you understand then why you were bad, what actually happened then?

Simone: Hm. *(indicating no)*

Interviewer: No?

Simone: Hm.

Interviewer: Hm?

Simone: I'd like to play a game that goes quickly.

Interviewer: I don't know anything that goes quickly. Couldn't we just talk a bit more?

Simone: Hm *(indicating no)*. I've got another idea. There's a shark *(points to a shelf)* there, isn't there? We could play with it a bit.

Interviewer: All right then, bring two or three toy animals you think you can play with over here.

Simone: And also the crocodile up there.

Interviewer: We're only just beginning to get to know a small piece of Simone. I've heard there's a bad Simone somewhere, then also a nice Simone, and he changes form ...

Simone: And someday even a religious Simone!

Interviewer: What is a religious person?

Simone: That I'm spiritual!

Interviewer: A spirit?

Simone: That I'm invisible.

Interviewer: Ah, so there's also an invisible Simone, and one who likes to confuse others and fluster them. But I could imagine that I could also sometimes be confusing for you too. So how do you get the nice, the bad and all the other Simones together under one hat?

Simone: I don't know yet either.

Interviewer: Yes, and that's confusing. Would you like to make another story with these *(the toy animals)*?

Simone: Yes, with you!

Interviewer: Yes.

Simone: You may go and get yourself one, I'll be these two, no, these three, and you be ... no I'll be these three, and you be these three.

Interviewer: I'll be these three, good; how does the story start then?

Simone: With a squirrel.

Interviewer: What?

Simone: With a squirrel and the crocodile.

Interviewer: So I'm the big crocodile and I'm hungry?

Simone: For me?

Interviewer: Hungry, I'd like to eat!

Simone: Me?

Interviewer: Whatever's there, I'd like to eat it.

Simone: Meat!

Interviewer: A squirrel if there's a squirrel there.

Simone: Catch me then!

Interviewer: Yes, I can try doing that, but the little animal is just much too fast for me, you know, I'm a really slow creature, but if I catch you I'll snap you up.

Simone: Do you know what?

Interviewer: No.

Simone: I'll give you some acorns!

Interviewer: That's good, I'll eat the acorns then.

Simone: Sorry, but that one's unripe ...

Interviewer: Yes, that was an unripe one, I didn't like it at all.

Simone: Hello, that's my friend.

Interviewer: Ah, that's Mr Shark, what's Mr Shark doing around here? I've never eaten sharks before, that's something I don't like so much.

Simone: And I don't much like eating crocodiles!

Interviewer: Aha, in that case we two must keep out of each other's way a bit.

Simone: No.

Interviewer: You can swim, I do sometimes too, but I can walk around, and you can't.

Simone: What?

Interviewer: Are you a squirrel?

Simone: Yes.

Interviewer: Ah!

Simone: No, I'm not a squirrel, I'm a skunk.

Interviewer: Ooh—a skunk! Then I'm getting quickly back in the water, I don't like them, not at all. If you're sprayed by a skunk, then you stink yourself, even when the skunk has gone ...

Simone: Hello—hey, hey ...!

Interviewer: Ah, now there's a little tiger cub, I think that would also taste good.

Simone: And I like you.

Interviewer: Yes, then I could ... *(scuffling play-fighting)*

Simone: (makes noises with his mouth).

Interviewer: Yes, with the tiger, we can play, it doesn't have to be eaten at all, that's a funny thing, ah here comes a small leopard now and I'd also like to play with the little tiger. You two will have fun together!

Simone: Shall we be friends?

Interviewer: Yes of course, but are there also some that aren't our friends?

Simone: Among the other animals?

Interviewer: Yes, how do the little tiger and the little leopard live?

Simone: Together!

Interviewer: Yes, but they'd also like to eat something.

Simone: Yes, but these two, not those two.

Interviewer: Aha, the hunger of these two is dangerous for those two.

Simone: But the crocodile eats them ...

Interviewer: Look now, ooh, a shark, oh we can't get in the water, that's not good, then we'd better go and get a squirrel.

Simone: I didn't need it, there, I'm in the water too.

Interviewer: Ah, that's not good, we can't get back out of the water now.

Simone: Now I'm back on the ...

Interviewer: Ah, but that's a skunk, that's not good at all.

Simone: (laughs)

Interviewer: Now, if we're hungry, we two ...

Simone: Change again into the squirrel!

Interviewer: Yes, a small squirrel would also be good.

Simone: Okay, then, a nut on the head!

Interviewer: Uh, nuts, that's not so good, there I must be careful it doesn't hurt. Nuts on the head, that's not for you, for leopards ...

Simone: But for me, always have a nut.

Interviewer: Well, I've never yet seen that, a shark that eats nuts, but anything is possible, but tell me now, we have a Simone who is sitting here, and he may also be a skunk, can you understand that? I don't understand that yet. Simone seems to be quite a complicated person.

Simone: I have ... that's a biblical name, Simone.

Interviewer: That's right, what else do you know then about Simone, the biblical one?

Simone: Hm, ah yes, I, Simone, carried the cross of Jesus up to the hill.

Interviewer: Yes, then you're actually a very strong person?

Simone: I would actually so like to be allowed to keep this squirrel!

Interviewer: I understand that—but it must stay here, unfortunately I can't give it to you to take away.

Simone: Who does it belong to then?

Interviewer: It belongs here in the room, you know, that belongs to other people who work here ...

Simone: Now you're making salami slices from it ...

Interviewer: Ah, now it's as if you wanted to stay with your squirrel-hunger, as you have a really proper squirrel-hunger ...

Simone: The squirrel is hungry?

Interviewer: No, you're hungry for the squirrel.

Simone: Yes.

Interviewer: Yes exactly, now I have to leave you alone with the hunger, just as the two *(tiger and crocodile)* are alone with their hunger right now ...

Simone: Okay!

Interviewer: The hunger ...

Simone: For the hunger you have ... meat!

Interviewer: Yes, but that's not fresh meat, that's old meat, I'd like to have fresh meat!

Simone: Okay, crocodile come ...

Interviewer: What's this?
Simone: Mm ...
Interviewer: What is it?
Simone: Can I look in your mouth for a moment?
Interviewer: Yes, but that's dangerous. For I have a really big mouth.
Simone: I'd just like to look at it.
Interviewer: What would you like to look at there?
Simone: To see if you have all your teeth.
Interviewer: Yes, they're big, and I've a lot of them, watch out.
Simone: Yes.
Interviewer: I can snap with them!
Simone: Yes, open your mouth.
Interviewer: Now I'm opening it.
Simone: (Makes biting noises)
Interviewer: ... just then I could still have escaped into the water—now we suddenly have a battle situation ...
Simone: Now we have fresh crocodile meat!
Interviewer: That's something else of course ... there we have ...
Simone: Rebirth, now I'm eating you up!
Interviewer: That's just being eaten up. Each one eats another.
Simone: But you've not played the lion yet.
Interviewer: No, the lion hasn't come at all yet. Watch out; now he's making a big sentence; he comes forward and says: I am the lion!
Simone: Retreating, I don't like lions at all, I'd much rather go back in the water.
Interviewer: That way is perhaps also good ...
Simone: And I'm also perhaps ...
Interviewer: Also right.
Simone: And I, I'll get on to the tree.
Interviewer: Good, but a lion is really all alone. A shark's also alone, he must look out so that something ...
Simone: There's a squirrel.
Interviewer: A squirrel?
Simone: Okay?
Interviewer: Yes, a squirrel, that's ...
Simone: Changing again into the skunk!
Interviewer: Oh, I don't like skunks at all, no, no, no ...!
Simone: Changing again into the shark!
Interviewer: Yes, sharks are in the water ...
Simone: I'm out of it now.
Interviewer: I've never seen that before, a shark that can walk around on land, that ...

Simone: Ciao, now I'm going to ... do you want to look at mine?

Interviewer: Hm?

Simone: Do you want to look at mine?

Interviewer: No, but you know, our time has now run out, we must say 'ciao' to the crocodile.

Simone: (arranges the animals in a row)

Interviewer: So, goodbye all you three.

Simone: Ciao.

Interviewer: Ciao. Simone made me realise that he can change form very quickly.

Simone: Only into animals.

Interviewer: Only into animals, but sometimes he doesn't know how he can bring together all the various 'Simone parts' that are there next to each other. Perhaps, Simone, that's a task for this time you're spending with us, for you to try to put all these parts together. So, now we'll go out and turn off the machine.

Simone: Er, I'd just like to look at something ...

Interviewer: We must stop now!

(Both leave the room together.)

Simone is then heard saying: the emergency number for the ambulance is 1112.

Interviewer: I've heard it: emergency!

References

Bürgin D. (1992): Kritzelzeichnungen als Landmarken im diagnostisch–therapeutischen Dialog mit Kindern und Jugendlichen [Squiggle drawings as landmarks in diagnostic–therapeutic dialogue with children and adolescents]. In: Hennig H./Fikentscher E./Rosendahl W. (ed.): Tiefenpsychologisch fundierte Psychotherapie mit dem Katathymen Bilderleben. HalleWittenberg: Martin Luther University.

Bürgin D. and Steck B. (2013): Indikation psychoanalytischer Psychotherapie bei Kindern, und Jugendlichen [Indication of psychoanalytic psychotherapy with children and adolescents]. Stuttgart: Klett-Cotta.

Notes

1 This is a reference to Winnicott's Squiggle game (1971). See also Bürgin 1992 and Bürgin and Steck 2013.

2 KPA = Kinderpsychiatrische Abteilung (child psychiatry department).

4 Anamnestic data and dates of hospitalisation periods

4.1 Family anamnesis

Simone's mother comes from a southern European country, lives apart from the child's father and has had no contact with him for several years now. The mother's father is said to have been an alcoholic who died prematurely following a short illness, while her mother had physically and mentally abused her children and had been unable to show any love. The mother's elder brother had died of an overdose in early adulthood. She herself had been repeatedly hospitalised for an eating disorder, depressions and suicidal tendencies, had grown up in care homes and foster families, and had had to repeat some years at school. She had suffered from stomach pains from eating disorders and repeatedly refused to attend school. As a pre-pubescent, she was diagnosed with *psycho-organic syndrome with hyperactivity*. After completing school, she began some studies that she broke off, and she later worked as a kitchen assistant. Various changes of residence were mentioned. Contact with her relatives had ceased. A year before Simone's birth, the mother made her first suicide attempt. In that year she got to know the child's father. The parents stayed together for a short period because of the pregnancy. But the child's father separated from her permanently once their son was 18 months old. Three years later they divorced. At the time of the interview, the mother was living with a partner who suffered from a severe chronic illness. She showed symptoms of bulimia. One year before the interview, she had been hospitalised in a psychiatric clinic because of a further suicide attempt and depressions. (She had been diagnosed with a borderline personality structure.) After the divorce, initially the father saw his son every two weeks. But the mother was convinced that when he was two years old her son had been physically mistreated and sexually abused by the father during the visiting days—a suspicion that could never be corroborated by the various authorities but finally led to the father breaking off contact with his son.

DOI: 10.4324/9781003304340-4

4.2 Personal anamnesis

The mother describes the pregnancy as unwanted. At first she had misinterpreted it as gastroenteritis and then later contemplated and tried to carry out an abortion with 'household remedies'. From the fourth month of pregnancy, she had suffered from contractions with bleeding, for which she was given pain-blocking medicines. In the middle of the pregnancy, she jumped into a river to rescue a child but probably also with the more or less conscious intention of instigating a premature birth or abortion. Finally, the baby was delivered by caesarean section because it was in the breech position. The infant suffered from atopic dermatitis. The mother suffered from great anxiety that her son would be disabled. Altogether the picture emerged—for the period of the pregnancy and the patient's birth—of a variously traumatic and emotionally deprived situation.

The child had shown no smile in response to a gaze in the third month and no stranger anxiety in the eighth month; at that time, however, he begun to beam at any person who took up contact with him. For eight and a half months, the boy was breastfed every half hour. He had begun early to develop his own words. At around 18 months, he had begun to walk and run seamlessly but had often fallen over. He had often hit himself. Even as a small child he had liked to play 'police and emergency lights' and always wanted to impose his own will. When he was two and half years old, the patient suffered from nightmares. The mother reported having always suffered from the fear of her child being stolen from her. She experienced his phase of defiance at the age of two years as extreme and described the fiercest power battles between her and her son. Simone was attending a play group with cerebrally paralysed children.

From his third year of life, the patient exhibited only a *minimal frustration tolerance* and *rather aggressive emotional outbursts.* At nursery school the contact with other children had become problematic. Simone had been bullied by the teacher and often been made to stand in front of the door or in the corner. He had often suffered from *stomach aches* and shown *poor concentration.*

In the first class, the *furious outbursts* and *impulsive behaviour* persisted. Simone attracted notice by his reduced attentiveness and day-dream-like absences. Soon after he started school, there was an investigation in the educational psychology service. A first attempt at therapy failed. Then he was *excluded* from the regular class partly because of increasing problems between the school directors and the mother. Then a paediatric assessment was carried out because of an uncertain psycho-organic syndrome. When he was six years old, a minor cerebral functional disturbance was ascertained in the patient by an electroencephalogram. This was followed by a placement in a *pedagogical children's ward* for two and a half months and then the attempt at an accompanying family support.

At the age of seven, Simone was diagnosed with a *severe sensorimotor developmental delay*. He quickly got exhausted and his concentration was very erratic. In well-structured situations with personal attention, however, he demonstrated good and interested collaboration. The mother regarded her son as a monster that wanted to harm her, constantly provoked her, could hardly be pacified, ran around, squealed and thrashed around. Insupportable states predominated at home.

Just after his seventh birthday, Simone was treated by the family doctor and given a *neuroleptic* because he had threatened to jump off the balcony and kill himself. Simone had already been expelled from the regular school. He had received individual teaching. The diagnosis at the time was: *acute decompensation of an attention deficit disorder with hyperactivity*. Shortly afterwards he was *taken into a university paediatric clinic* as an in-patient (diagnosis: attention deficit hyperactivity disorder, reactive attachment disorder, social behaviour disorder, depression). Soon he was transferred and received as in-patient in the *children's and adolescents' psychiatric clinic*. On admission the mother proved to be completely exhausted, helpless and extremely fearful. She could no longer tolerate the situation and could no longer get through to her son. She saw him as a kind of devil.

Simone himself made appropriate contact with the new caregivers and liked playing with the *ambulance*. He was attached to the mother's partner and sought bodily contact with him. The *mother showed a tendency to projective distortions*, presented herself as extremely tough and demanding but was actually very gentle and emotional. She seemed to be absolutely desperate and at the end of her tether.

Test-based psychological examination: a clever, charming, expectant boy who demands attention. Provocative, cheeky or denigrating remarks. Rather poorly distanced. Immediately sounds out the counterpart's boundaries and tests the framework. With consistent direction, Simone seems to be easily motivated. He collaborates willingly and obediently but soon loses interest. He has only a reduced capacity for concentration, low stamina and an increased exhaustibility. Makes lots of excuses. Has a wide vocabulary, age-appropriate understanding of language, unclear articulation. Graphomotorically retarded. IQ between 85 und 111, which means: average intellectual ability. Major emotional oscillations. Depressive, helpless and lacking orientation. Anxieties about failure, to the point of resignation. Overplays everything in a compensatory way by clowning around. If his own needs remain unmet or unheard, Simone resorts to suicide threats. He feigns an unshakeable self-assurance but is in reality a small, shy boy, extremely hungry for relationships, who quickly feels insulted and rejected, makes clingy attempts at closer contact, reveals a disturbed distance-regulation and expresses poorly controlled wishes for contact. Many things can shatter his equilibrium, disturb his pseudo-stability and quickly lead to aggressive behaviour.

At the department: Simone behaves hyperactively in manifold ways. But his sadness quickly becomes perceptible. He exhibits problems with closeness–distance regulation. He makes contact through cheekiness and insults. The conversational thread is therefore soon torn again. No major noticeable features in his thinking. Already on the first evening, some physically aggressive escalations resulting from not accepting boundaries.

After one month of in-patient treatment: the mother joins a sect and from then on experiences her son on the one hand as a beast, on the other as an affectionate and charming boy. Simone's behaviour is characterised by rapid mood swings, furious outbursts, lack of distance, reduced endurance and concentration, as well as high distractibility. He tries by means of negative or sexualised behaviour to gain attention, but he also has a capacity to enter relationships affectionately and openly. His sense of self-worth is low. Everything is divided into 'good' or 'bad'. The EEG is unremarkable.

When he is only just eight years old, after about half a year of in-patient treatment, Simone behaves in an *extraordinarily destructive* way, destroying some furniture. At school as well, he appears increasingly *aggressive-rejecting, and verbally extremely insulting.* He plays destructive war games with 'funny cripples', is then 'disabled himself', falls over in a faint and 'dies'. Or in play he takes over the role of the devil and wants to be hit.

Some time later he becomes *emotionally very difficult to reach.* He appears indifferent and provocative at the same time, intensely seeks boundaries and needs sedation. Now he is as nice as can be at home, and wildly aggressive, defiant and demanding at the department. Or he plays the clown, is hyperactive and exaggerated. The theme of sexuality is in the foreground—as an activator. At school he will not get involved in any work, demands a great deal of attention and is constantly provocative.

In the week of the interview, he attracts attention by an endless need for communication, although he is really well integrated into the group. From time to time, there is a sign that he wants to learn something. He sticks to agreements better. But repeatedly there are fits of rage, he destroys objects, is fascinated by war and weapons, dresses as a woman, calls for boundaries and looks for a father figure.

Over the next two months (still hospitalised) he can play in a structured way. His frustration tolerance seems to have improved, but he is still behaving provocatively, kicking other children and knocking them down. Overall though he keeps to agreements and tolerates rebukes. At school he works with more concentration.

The mother complains about major problems at her workplace and about financial problems. In conflicts between the mother and her partner, Simone takes the blame on to himself and willingly gets scorched. He often behaves dominantly towards weaker children. He still likes dressing as a girl and looks for a father figure. Meek as a lamb at the weekends, he comes back happy and chatty. Meanwhile the mother has been going to therapy of her own.

There are continual aggressive outbursts with kicking and hitting. Sometimes he denies himself. 'No' is then the key word. During phases of quarrelling he scarcely keeps to agreements, does not enter into conversations and cannot reflect.

Just before leaving he speaks, having set off a fire alarm, for the first time about his father and a secret, but at the same time behaves as if none of this had anything to do with him. Very arrogantly, Simone throws around some incredibly angry insults. In many quarrels he hits out at objects, but he soon calms down and shows increasing attempts at integrating bad and good self-parts.

5 Commentaries by the group participants

After detailed scrutiny of the volume and long conversations about the various views and basic assumptions we encountered, we decided that each participant should look at the volume and the transcript again alone and then write down his own impressions against the background of his own basic assumptions, so that both the similarities and the differences would become visible. The four commentaries were discussed again afterwards to explain anything that was unclear and to deepen the mutual understanding amid all the differences.

5.1 Commentary 1 (Dieter Bürgin)

5.1.1 Observations on the use of 'squiggles'

General: in the intrapsychic realm of a human being, affects, thoughts and images arise. They all go to create the prevailing appearance of a meaningful dialogue (see Faimberg, 2019). A meaningful dialogue is a precondition for a diagnostic and therapeutic process with a child and an adolescent. It is sustained by both partners in the dialogue.

Winnicott's squiggle game is one form this dialogue can take; it is a way of 'making and staying in contact' with the patient's conscious and unconscious personality components. What happens in this game can only be elucidated against the background of a theory of how a relationship develops. In the commonly 'held' transitional space, the child remains protected, trust develops and a specific atmosphere arises that Winnicott called the 'sacred moment'.

A child or adolescent, if an appropriate opportunity arises, expresses his current problems and/or emotional conflicts or set of tensions within the circumscribed situation of the professional contact. In this way there is already a mass of 'material' available for a psychodynamic diagnosis and for a possible psychoanalytic treatment. In a therapeutic consultation, the

DOI: 10.4324/9781003304340-5

patient quickly comes to sense that an attempt is being made to understand him and he may experience a special kind of communication at a meaningful level. Sometimes dramatic changes ensue; sometimes the door only opens a crack. The quality and significance of such a dialogue becomes a means of assessing the neediness, capacity and motivation for allowing oneself to enter an analytic process, forming a picture of the present anxieties, defences and readiness for transference and recognising how and in what way a patient can make use of an analyst.

In this 'acting', the analyst divides himself into two different figures: on the one hand he is the one who is doing something, and on the other he is the one who observes himself and finally reflects on the product. Something similar applies for the child or a young person. The patient also, as someone who is drawing (i.e. engaged in activity or amplifying a squiggle) has another self available that observes the active self and that—often critically or doubtingly like the analyst—tries to observe the origination of what is happening.[1] It repeatedly becomes clear that the active person becomes frustrated more quickly than the one who is observing.

The methodology of the squiggle drawings according to Winnicott (1973) is therefore both a diagnostic and a therapeutic aid for building and maintaining a dialogue. The image that comes to light corresponds to a visual realisation of the joint creations taking place in the transitional spaces. This leads on to language and to more pictures. Often the creations are mysterious at first. Sooner or later a wish emerges in both protagonists to establish a meaning for what has arisen. The more a representation gains a specific meaning, the more it becomes separated from other possible representations. In instances where suddenly the possibility of a connection is seen, this acts as a moment of revelation (Kentridge, 2017, p. 67). The more peripheral ideas automatically recede into the background, but, if adequately observed, they can create entirely relevant meanings.

By telling stories about the (jointly) made drawings, children and adolescents amplify the iconographic and scenic communications, problems and conflicts with narrative elements. If the child remains protected in the transitional space created in that way, which is bridged with dialogue, a specific atmosphere develops that contains the opportunity for an encounter on a newly created level. Blocked development can be relaxed or—in the ideal case—transformed into a continuation of the development process. The child himself gains an insight into what psychoanalytic work could be like. The analytic psychotherapist is strongly challenged. For he is directly drawn into the creations with the conscious and unconscious parts of his personality. So he must not only act, speak and reflect but also make rapid and deep identifications and dis-identifications with the patient. An especially precise verification of his own components and those of the counter-transference is indispensable, as otherwise there is a danger of one's own projections undermining the patient's defence.

Stories of children/adolescents about the jointly made squiggle drawings offer a possibility of verbalising interventions and interpretations based on this material (a level of displacement) before they are brought directly into connection with the transference/countertransference level. The squiggle game is therefore not a therapeutic technique but a helpful means of building and maintaining a dialogue that is enjoyably playful but painful and deeply serious at the same time.

On the theory: The blank paper is awaiting marks and lines that we have to apply to discover form and meanings. We are then simultaneously producers, observers, explainers and interpreters. "We try to extract meaning from the world by constructing it from different fragments", i.e. we do not simply receive the world as it comes towards us (Kentridge, 2017, p. 28). It is sought for drawing—a kind of membrane between the world and the paper—then taken apart and finally reassembled. In drawing, it encounters a sheet of paper with a specific texture and quality, which also help to determine the drawing. Materials therefore also change thoughts. Drawing is thinking in a material form, a way of finding meaning in the material. Images undergo a kind of migration when they travel from one form to another (ibid., p. 41). In this way, drawing becomes a meaning-generating activity, as it constructs meanings from different elements (p. 43). Because of their many possible meanings, the drawings also allow a space of ambiguity to arise; they open up provisional spaces (p. 47).

What happens to make an image arise rather than a thought? The drawing becomes something 'taking us from what we know to an image, a site, an insight we did not know we had' (Kentridge, 2014, p. 22). 'Something we don't know that we know. Something we can recognise without knowing' (Kentridge, 2014, p. 18). There is 'a drawing waiting to be made' (p. 30), although we have freedom of action as to whether we want to enter into it or not; 'there is something on the paper which triggers the recognition of [something] in us' (p. 18). What comes to us from outside meets us—i.e. what comes from inside—halfway. 'The drawing becomes a meeting point, but also a threshold where the outside world meets us' (p. 18). We stand in the middle of two realities. Light and shade form patterns and produce shared images that are ready to have an effect on the observer. There is a 'need for the darkness, for shadow, to be present for anything to be visible' (p. 45).

Obviously, there is a striving beyond language and logic (i.e. the secondary process) to reach meanings through the pathways of the primary process. Freedom and power, as well as insight and finding nothing, are entangled in a knot and may not find a goal for a long time. Something happens through the observation and assembly of intermediate spaces and gaps. In principle, however, no logical connection can usually be found between clearly definable external points and new meanings or forms. 'We are caught between wanting to send ourselves out and to hold back, to call back, to annul and obliterate so many traces and acts' (pp. 24–25), i.e. to make them unsaid, unremembered and 'unhappened'.

We learn 'in the gaps, in the leaps to complete an image ... we perform a generative act of constructing the shape' (p. 29). The 'very leanness of the illusion pushes us to complete the recognition' (p. 29). We repeatedly encounter configurations in which a child or adolescent who wanted to create an image of himself had had this forced on him from outside.

Confused thinking is not linear; one thought does not follow another and there is no directed stream of consciousness. Instead, one thought overflows somewhere into the other for as long as it takes for one thought to finally take the lead and set a direction. Often we find the physical world stands in for ideas and representations that we unconsciously carry inside. Through sensory perception, we invite the external world into our internal world, where it appears in fragmented form. Intrapsychically we order, combine and modify sometimes contradictory elements into a new whole, by adapting them to each other. For we are under pressure to give meaning to what is perceived. This new whole, a reconstruction, is then shifted into the external world in the form of drawings, products, texts and so on (Kentridge, 2019).

Images make it possible to observe things together and next to each other, until the decision emerges as to which elements are the most important. Are we like a porous membrane that receives all the projections directed at us and simultaneously sends these continuously itself? 'A drawing is a membrane between the world coming toward us and our projected understanding of the world, a negotiation between ourselves and that which is outside' (Kentridge, 2014, p. 76). Between the inner and the outer look, the projections occurring from inside and from outside, the ego functions partly as a membrane that receives the energy flowing in from both sides and—anticipating a potential collision—corresponds to the inner 'pressure of the material to be something else' (p. 67), so that by bringing together a multiplicity of unknown variables, forms, images, ideas or stories can be developed.

Everything is subject to transformation based on internal and external forces. The internal forces press outward in a violent movement, i.e. from inside something grows out that has an effect externally on the form, changes it, and finally by means of perception, i.e. having turned back, takes up the changed thing again and so finds a way to itself in a new form. 'An image [has] to sediment itself until the picture [is] thick with time' (p. 105).

This giving over to the medium is crucial. Allowing a space for the medium to lead, giving yourself over to the play itself. Playing not in the sense of following rules known in advance ... Not a random activity but giving yourself over to what the activity provokes.

(pp. 106–107)

In the end-product of the squiggling, two psyches (or two people) have succeeded in turning different things, i.e. their own and a stranger's, in a unified, illusory perspective that is shared, constructively paraphrased, into a whole. Apparently unconnected unities, under the pressure of relational and developmental coherence, are brought as free-floating fragments into a specific connection, which triggers similar processes in the psyche and the participating protagonists' capacities for speaking and thinking. The seemingly aimless shaping effects a change in what is defensively stagnating and allows the beginning of a flowing movement. The conscious renunciation of judging what is initially meaningless creates space for a free development of images, ideas, feelings or associations. In what has arisen jointly, parts of us are revealed 'that we neither expressed nor knew, until we saw them' (p. 128).

The patient presents us with an enigma for which he has so far found no better solution. 'NOT knowing the answer to the riddle opens all the possibilities and different possible answers' (pp. 136–137). By our attitude of helpfulness to the patient, however, we convey that we are not persuaded that his way of understanding the enigma that exists inside him is the only possible one. 'The riddle with the answer leaves behind the secondary riddle, of that which does not have an answer' (p. 137). The disappearance of the Sphinx after the enigma was solved by Oedipus only cleared the scene for many new enigmas.

In taking the journey into the unknown with a squiggle dialogue, both protagonists are brought into connection with the other's immeasurable differentness (and also with the parts in himself with which contact is hardly ever made). An approach both inwards and outwards ensues. The need to assemble the emerging fragments into a whole form intensifies. The discrepancy between this energy and the defensive incapacity to recognise how or why this should be done constitutes the force that revolves around an unknown centre. This involves a movement between potentiality and nothing, the frontier traffic between the membranes of what is uncertain in ourselves and what is uncertain in the other. We also feel the anxiety that with every decision in every conclusive arrival of an image or a thought, all other images or thoughts would be prohibited. This causes a tendency for order to dissolve into disorder and likewise an inclination to develop something—with an injection of energy—ordered from what is unordered. 'The meaning is always a construction, a projection, not an edifice—something to be made, not simply found' (2014, p. 185).

Squiggles and basic assumptions: at least two actual people take part in a dialogue but an infinite number of figures out of relational representations sing along with its tune. The establishment of a transitional space that belongs to neither one nor the other person but is used by both (in potentially different ways) as well as by the analytic setting make it possible to use the creations that arise in it playfully, to allow preconscious contents of an affective, cognitive, creative and transgenerational kind to appear figuratively and also to some extent verbally. In this way a psychoanalytic process is constituted in a micro-format that can be used diagnostically and therapeutically. The video-recording of this event—through the repeated and shared observation/listening to the notes made and in the shared exchange of the respective partners in conversation—allows all the participants' basic assumptions that have emerged to be retroactively elucidated.

5.1.2 Observations on basic assumptions and unconscious fantasies

The question quickly arises of course as to whether *basic assumptions* are not in fact the same as *unconscious fantasies*. Before we try to address some thoughts on this question, the concept of unconscious fantasies, as it emerged with Freud and was developed by Melanie Klein, should be briefly considered in more detail. As early as The Interpretation of Dreams, the concept appears as a background structure that is responsible for symptom-formation:

> Thus some of the activities whose successful performance in dreams excited astonishment are now no longer to be attributed to dreams but to unconscious thinking ... those representations are the product of certain unconscious phantasies ... which find expression not only in dreams but also in hysterical phobias and other symptoms
>
> (Freud, 1900, p. 613)

Only one year later Freud links unconscious fantasies with the 'déjà vu'-experience:

> Those psychical processes which according to my observations are alone responsible for the explanation of *'déjà vu'*—namely, unconscious phantasies—are still generally neglected by psychologists even to-day.
>
> (Freud, 1901, p. 265)

Some years later, Freud considers fantasies in connection with daydreams and the possibility of making these conscious. Daydreams in the sense of fantasies with the potential to become conscious exist both unconsciously and consciously. If they have been repressed, they can become pathological, i.e. be expressed in symptoms and attacks. 'In favourable circumstances, the subject can still capture an unconscious phantasy of this sort in consciousness' (Freud, 1908a, p. 159).

Then Freud posed the question of whether unconscious fantasies are a primary or a secondary phenomenon:

> Unconscious phantasies have either been unconscious all along and have been formed in the unconscious; or—as is more often the case—they were once conscious phantasies, day-dreams, and have since been purposely forgotten and have become unconscious through 'repression' ... Now an unconscious phantasy has a very important connection with the subject's sexual life.
>
> (p. 160)

And he reformulated the connection between unconscious fantasies and symptom formation:

> Hysterical symptoms are nothing other than unconscious phantasies brought into view through 'conversion' ... The technique of psychoanalysis enables us in the first place to infer from the symptoms what those unconscious phantasies are ... it has been found that the content of the hysteric's unconscious phantasies corresponds completely to the situations in which satisfaction is consciously obtained by perverts.
>
> (pp. 160–161)

Unconscious fantasies probably comprise an 'endeavour to find expression, the relationship of the phantasies to the symptoms is not simple, but on the contrary, complicated in many ways' (p. 162). Symptoms, as realisations of unconscious fantasies, show

> that there are many symptoms where the uncovering of a sexual phantasy (or of a number of phantasies, one of which, the most significant and the earliest, is of a sexual nature) is not enough to bring about a resolution of the symptoms. To resolve it one has to have two sexual phantasies, of which one has a masculine and the other a feminine character. Thus, one of these phantasies springs from a homosexual impulse.
>
> (p. 164)

Finally, Freud also re-emphasised the rapid *changeability* of unconscious fantasies:

> We must not suppose that the products of this imaginative activity—the various phantasies, castles in the air and daydreams—are stereotyped or unalterable. On the contrary, they fit themselves in to the subject's shifting impressions of life, change with every change in his situation, and receive from every fresh active impression what might be called a 'date-mark'. The relation of a phantasy to time is in general very important. We may say that it hovers, as it were, between three times—the three moments of time which our ideation involves. Mental work is linked to some current impression, some provoking occasion in the present which has been able to arouse one of the subject's major wishes. From there it harks back to a memory of an earlier experience (usually an infantile one) in which this wish was fulfilled; and it now creates a situation relating to the future which represents a fulfilment of the wish. What it thus creates is a day-dream or phantasy, which carries about it traces of its origin from the occasion which provoked it and from the memory. Thus past, present and future are strung together, as it were, on the thread of the wish that runs through them.
>
> (1908b, pp. 146–147)

Throughout the *Freud–Klein debates of 1943–1944*, the concept of unconscious fantasy and the corresponding implications and consequences were in the foreground. Unconscious fantasies, as representations of earlier libidinous and aggressive relationships to inner and outer objects or partial objects that are initially based on bodily experiences, were the chief bone of contention.

The earliest, completely unconscious fantasies are constructed from partial objects, averbal transferred elements, purely primary-process processed sensations, thought processes, archaic affects (greed, envy, elimination) and/or genetic components. Melanie Klein expressed the conviction,

> that unconscious, primitive phantasies—initially of receiving and expelling—are connected from the outset of life with bodily processes and drive impulses that are directed at an object. Primitive object relations are the content of unconscious phantasies. Through these first psychic mechanisms of introjection and projection, an inner world of internalised objects is constructed—both good objects connected with the life drive of the love of the child and bad persecutory objects that represent the death drive. These internal objects, which as part of

the ego form the early superego, are in constant exchange with real objects, being influenced by them, but also colouring how they are perceived.

(Cycon R., 1994, p. x, translated quotation)

Melanie Klein herself argued that *very early fantasies probably always remain unconscious*, especially if they are aggressive in nature:

normally we only get comparatively faint indications of the small child's impulses to destroy its object. What we see are only derivatives of its phantasies in that connection. That the child should express its intensely sadistic impulses towards its external objects in such a weakened form becomes more intelligible if we assume that the extravagant phantasies which arise in a very early stage of its development never become conscious at all. It should, moreover, be remembered that the stage of ego-development in which such phantasies occur is a very early one and that the child's relations to reality are as yet very much influenced by its imaginative life. A further reason may be found in its inferiority in size and strength to the adult and in its biologically determined dependence on him; for we see how much more strongly it manifests its destructive instincts towards inanimate things, small animals, and so on.

(Klein, 1932, pp. 212–213)

Four years later Klein again referred to *unconscious fantasies* as the *most primitive activity* of the psyche:

Analytic work has shown that babies of a few months of age certainly indulge in phantasy-building. I believe that this is the most primitive mental activity and that phantasies are in the mind of the infant almost from birth. It would seem that every stimulus the child receives is immediately responded to by fantasies, the unpleasant stimuli, including mere frustration, by phantasies of an aggressive kind, the gratifying stimuli by those focusing on pleasure.

(Klein, 1936, p. 290)

The baby's impulses and feelings are accompanied by a kind of mental activity which I take to be the most primitive one: that is phantasy-building, or more colloquially, imaginative thinking ... Such primitive fantasising is the earliest form of the capacity which later develops into the more elaborate workings of the imagination.

(Klein, 1936, p. 308)

Finally, she also emphasises the connection between early infantile uncon-scious fantasies and *omnipotent thinking*:

> The early phantasies which go along with the baby's feelings are of various kinds ... Pleasant phantasies, however, also accompany actual satisfaction; and destructive phantasies go along with frustration and the feelings of hatred which this arouses ... the baby feels that what he desires in his phantasies has really taken place; that is to say he feels that he *has really destroyed* the object of his destructive impulses, and is going on destroying it: this has extremely important consequences for the development of his mind. The baby finds support against these fears in omnipotent phantasies of a restoring kind: that too has extremely important consequences for his development ... In my view, these basic conflicts profoundly influence the course and the force of the emotional lives of grown-up individuals.
>
> (1936, pp. 308–309)

It is likely that *fantasies* are also imagined fulfilments of unsatisfied drive wishes that primarily revolve around separation, the primal scene, castra-tion and seduction. But they also portray at the earliest stage *schemata of innate unities* (Stern), even before the thinking apparatus has developed (Bion, 1962), and later form the basic material for dreams, for fantasying and finally also for the whole primary process of thinking.

It seems highly probable that unconscious fantasies, depending on the respective drive activity, the wishes arising from it, the quality of object relationships, corresponding frustrations or satisfactions and not least defences, are also being shaped. These are therefore both products of intrin-sic maturation, and results of the ego's extrinsic activity, i.e. perceptions or interactive experiences with the external world (development), which are constantly being further differentiated.

The older an individual becomes, the more important the component of experience becomes in the quality of unconscious fantasies. For the ego goes through a scarcely hormonalised phase in early and late childhood (infantile sexuality), the period of a relatively fast hormonalisation in adoles-cence and hormone reduction in the 'menopause' (quicker in women, slower in men). In these time periods, very different hormonal effects occur on the brain. Accordingly, different drive and need intensities appear, as well as changed forms of ego-functioning. With it, all the experiential qualities play a part in dealing with the external world in the elaboration of ever new and from then on also old unconscious, preconscious and conscious fantasies. In end-less diversity and continuing variability, as the result of central intrapsychic activity, a repertoire of unconscious fantasies arises that finally influences the individual's own thinking and also interpersonal activities.

Basic assumptions also (according to my basic assumption) undergo a development in the course of the life cycle. They arise in the fantasy space by being raised, abstracted and prototyped to a higher and next-higher level of conceptualisation. Initially they constitute an overarching aggregated result of the fusion of unconscious fantasies. In the course of development, however, they are increasingly modified by ever richer experiences (i.e. by inclusion of the perceptual apparatus and perceptual processing). Nevertheless, the verification of the first outlines of basic assumptions within the ego's complex everyday functions, in developing relationships and also in the affects, gives rise to a possibility of modification. For these must have proved themselves in the understanding and intrapsychic classification of experiences over a certain period of time and acquired a certain relevance. Basic assumptions also form and in this way differentiate the space in which further unconscious fantasies can arise. By being tested in the mastery of everyday life, they take on an increasing number of ego-structuring tasks.

If the more visual-concrete unconscious fantasies, because of their effortless displaceability and rapid changeability, have a strong dynamism that must be 'maintained' if it is not to overflow (which can sometimes occur by means of the basic assumptions), then the more abstract basic assumptions show a much greater stability, uniformity on the time axis and a deep influence on the ordering, understanding and conceptualising ego-functions. Basic assumptions therefore also change during the life cycle and assume increasingly complex tasks within the ego-structure.

Basic assumptions acquire a pathogenic quality if they stay the same in unchanged form over decades, i.e. if they are not deepened in any way by new experiential worlds, changed ego structures or new relationship and defence configurations in the course of life, but as unconscious assumptions remain effective in the same way as at the time they were formed. Long-term experiences in psychoanalytic processes, which allow transformations, are mostly also connected with gradual, ever deeper reformulations of conscious and unconscious basic assumptions (and so of course also of unconscious, preconscious and conscious fantasies). Basic assumptions may never have become conscious; we then refer to primary unconscious basic assumptions. Or they have been repressed or displaced by other forms of defence into the unconscious; then we refer to secondary unconscious basic assumptions. The reactivation of primary or secondary unconscious basic assumptions in the transference and their processing—including with the aid of the countertransference, i.e. in the relationship and their clarification in the analytic process—could represent the place at which small-step, structurally effective changes can ensue.

The more splitting mechanisms a child, adolescent or adult person uses, the more he divides the self into a henceforth averagely functioning part and a radically changed part. In the latter, many basic assumptions about his own person, his own relationships and his own being are completely changed. As Bollas observed: 'We are governed by thousands of unthought known axioms that we never think because they formed before we had concepts with which to think them' (Bollas, 2015, pp. 181–182). If preconscious basic assumptions are formulated, they lose their affiliation to the unthought known and are 'subjected to thought' (p. 183).

In the analytic process, most personal basic convictions are worked through. The changing of the psyche by infantile distorted or psychotic basic assumptions brings about structural changes. The attempt to help to change the mental structures can be made by first working through those basic assumptions that triggered a symptom formation. The totality of an analyst's basic-assumptions determines how he listens, to what his empathy relates and how he can fundamentally present himself as a person. With appropriate understanding and adequate regard on his part, interpretations based on the patient's worked-out basic assumptions are no longer experienced by the latter as a danger. It can then be observed how in a transitional stage the patient moves back and forth 'between the analysand's former unconscious assumptions and new ones emerging from the work of psychotherapy' (p. 184). The more pronounced a disturbance, the greater the need to transform the corresponding basic assumptions by interpretation. 'Once the therapist has analysed several of the core assumptions, then it is as if the mind recalibrates other disturbed axioms, and an endogenous intrapsychic change takes place' (p. 186). Such changes become recognisable when an individual's thinking, emotions, fantasies and behaviour are newly directed with the aid of changed assumptions and no longer by the original basic assumption.

5.1.3 The interview

I would like to consider the interview from the perspective of what basic assumptions we connect with the psychoanalytic setting. The fundamental rule brings about a change in the patient's orientation towards his inner world. It is based on the acceptance by both sides of an asymmetric division of tasks. As an analytic basic assumption, the idea exists that in an interpersonal communication that is not goal-directed and does not proceed by the usual communicative rules (namely to say everything that comes into one's mind), the apparently confused processes internal to the patient's psyche are determined by a functional matrix and structure and interactional dynamics (in terms of content, emotion, the drives, defences and superego) at the basis of the psyche. Similarly, in that encounter but above all also a new one, relational representations from the past are activated, in the hope that these might also prove themselves in the new situation as guiding principles and might be appropriate. Timeless events from the primary process are brought into a temporal sequence by the rules that govern the verbal. The sequence of processes therefore becomes information for the analyst himself.

The interview begins—in a situation that contains a more or less clear challenge to self-disclosure—with the interviewer's wish for them to get to know each other and to discover why the patient has been hospitalised, as well as with the patient's request to draw and above all to remain hidden ('But people are well hidden there') and to encounter the given situation with the defence configuration of a role-reversal (Interviewer: 'And who would you look at then?' Simone: 'You ... Why don't we do it the other way round'?) The theme of the reflecting, one-way mirror is introduced by the patient. Simone also uses the means of coercion of the counterpart into a projective identification as a first transference movement. The counterpart—slightly distorting the situation—is experienced as someone who would like to confuse the patient. The interviewer thus becomes a figure from the patient's world of representations. He tries to form a picture of whether Simone is also in a position to take back this projection. (Interviewer: 'if you make sure the other person is not coming out anymore, then you can stay under a magic cloak. But that could mean you're actually very afraid someone might discover you'). Simone expresses very clearly that he is reliant for the further course of the encounter on knowing who his counterpart is. (Simone: ... 'To know who you are!') It would be bad for him if he encountered no resonance or no sense of being perceived by the other (Simone: 'When people keep not answering me').

Simone wants to draw, and the interviewer offers a drawing game (squiggles), but Simone gets his way with 'let's draw, let's draw'. He gradually forms a first narrative that constitutes an answer to the interviewer's question (as to why he has been hospitalised): a car with an emergency man and siren drives to a crashed vehicle from the children's and adolescents' psychiatric department (in which Simone is hospitalised) because a child needs help. (Interviewer: 'Do you think it could be that Simone is actually telling me he may urgently need help?' Simone: 'Urgently?' (shakes his head). Interviewer: 'Not so urgently? But all the same?' Simone: 'I think so too!'

In the meantime, Simone has obviously reassured himself that he can dare to enter the dialogue and use the counterpart as an extension of his psyche (one of the interviewer's basic assumptions). He begins to shape the flow of his communications in a shared transitional space (another of the interviewer's basic assumptions).

The picture emerges of a surface of water (waves) whirled up by a hurricane with a big fish and a small fish under it. The hurricane abates on one side. An intervention by the interviewer, who refers to Simone's stormy times with his mother (Interviewer: 'do you think we could say Simone had perhaps gone through some very stormy times with his Mummy?'), is first rejected, then accepted by the patient. Now a series of further drawings is added to the first: a pelican that wants to eat the fish appears (threat). (Simone: 'It wants to catch the fish'), but then also a man with a gun who protects the fish. He can put his head inside the wall. Because they can go a long way down and then a long way back up again, the fish find escape routes (Simone: 'and they can get to the other side of the sea; the fish don't have to experience the threatening danger; they can get through there. But they have to go a long way down … and then a long way up, as far as they have to go down'). The interviewer introduces a fox. Afterwards Simone wants his pencil and uses it to draw a fox's den.

Suddenly there is some treasure (Simone: 'And he can't get through it any more … because there's some treasure he wants to dig out with a spade, look now—we have a spade'). It becomes dangerous for the fox and the fish (Simone: 'Now it's getting a bit dangerous for the fox!'). By eating a lot, the fish turn into predator fish, into sharks with many rows of teeth (Simone is going through a change of teeth for the second dentition). A skull becomes an ambiguous symbol: it represents something eaten or possibly saved, but it is also a sign of some suffering having been caused to the shark (Interviewer: 'Ah, it's been drawn on, and does the shark have a plaster there?'. Simone: 'Yes, because someone's hurt it'. The fox wants to get the treasure but cannot at first because he cannot get through the water. Meanwhile a certainty has also arisen that the fish are a mother and child (Simone: 'That's its child, it already has a few fins on its back, but they're already long, look'). It appears that Simone has already thought up a continuing story that is arranged on various loose pages. A 'blue gun' for protection appears that is used to shoot (Interviewer: 'Does it continue there, or does it go on to a new page?' Simone: 'A new one will do. Then he's holding a blue gun, he's also shooting with it, look now … You know, that's the fox's mate there, that's the other side of the mountain, and now he's dug a huge hole there for the pelican so he can get through, and there the pelican has made just as a big a hole, look!'). The fox and the pelican manage to get through a hole to the treasure. The fox (introduced by the interviewer) joins with the sharks (Simone-products). In the end the sharks can escape. In the sequence of events Simone tells a story about the persistent threatening and rescue of a mother with a child with an increasing level of aggression. It seems as if Simone wants to use his counterpart to communicate to him a kind of symbolised brief biography. With dream-like scene changes, both the defensive and the drive impulses are taken into account.

A new theme comes to the fore: children's birth but after the mother's death. It remains unclear whether this is possible for both sexes. Simone would like to take away the pictures (Simone: 'Can I take this drawing away with me?') and must tolerate the refusal, as he obviously does. The new mother and her new child turn first into swordfish, then hammerhead sharks (Simone: 'And they've been made smaller, look, now the smaller one has got bigger and now it's had a small baby, do you know why?' Interviewer: 'No'. Simone: 'Because the mother has died, and that was the girl'). Finally, the repetitive theme of perpetual transmutation and variation appears.

Do we encounter the repetition compulsion here as a defence or as a new beginning? It seems to contain the wish to become 'nicer' as something that is possible through 'further development' (Interviewer: 'I would actually still be interested in what you did in order not to be bad any more'. Simone: 'Developed further!').

5.1.4 Playing with the toy animals

The change of scene that follows leads from the drawing game into playing with the toy animals, in which the interviewer as a person is even more strongly included. Simone registers there various self-components (e.g. the 'spiritual' Simone), his curiosity and also the wish to be invisible. (Simone to the crocodile): 'Can I look in your mouth for a moment?' Interviewer: 'Yes, but that's dangerous. For I have a really big mouth'. Simone: 'I'd just like to look at it'. Interviewer: 'What would you like to look at there?' Simone: 'To see if you have all your teeth'). The mouth cavity (the sharks' rows of teeth, the patient's change of teeth), i.e. the place where words also come out, seems to be of particular interest.

The themes here are hunger and eating, i.e. oral-libidinal (hunger also in the sense of longing for) and oral-aggressive strivings (eating up), but also anal-aggressive impulses (skunk). Interactively there is an enjoyable scuffling by the animals (and so symbolically also the two protagonists), which culminates in the patient wanting to be friends with the counterpart (Simone: 'Shall we be friends?'). Amid playful eating orgies Simone invents rebirth. Instead of eating each other, they can eat nuts. Again, Simone expresses the wish to take something specific with him, but he tolerates the refusal well here too. Transformation through constant further development is championed by the patient. But he can face up to the confrontation with the fact that it will be difficult to integrate into a whole all the various self-components (including that of Christ's crucifer and the wish to be invisible). In the doorway as he goes out, Simone mentions—as if incidentally in passing, but still again drawing attention to urgent need—the emergency phone number of the medical services!

5.1.5 Concluding remarks

According to the basic assumption that a patient must test out whether he can 'use' the psychoanalytic counterpart and in Winnicott's sense deploy him for his development, it can be said that Simone has done this with the interviewer in a deeper way. He has shown that, after initial hesitation, he could allow a loop-like 'emotional flow' towards the interviewer and back, which, modified by complex, magical-omnipotent defensive activity, could become the vehicle of preconscious 'meaningful material'. His creative capacity, under the given living conditions, to maintain and to shape the hunger for a relationship is considerable. Despite being strongly drawn into their joint activities, the interviewer has managed to maintain the analytic position. Both were able together—both creatively and in the flow of meaning—to carry out something like 'analytic work' in reciprocal relatedness. In the interview a shared third could arise. This (which is another of this author's basic assumptions) forms a progressive, development-fostering medium.

5.2 Commentary 2 (Anna Wyler von Ballmoos)

5.2.1 Introductory remarks

What are my basic assumptions in dealing with clinical material, and how do these basic assumptions shape the form and manner in which I hear, see, receive and understand the 'material'?

I hear, see and read about the events and try as a first exercise to stay with my own basic assumptions specific to me, of which I am conscious, which I have developed as a human being and adopted as a psychoanalyst. This way of proceeding enables me to receive the events in this description in a way that is familiar to me but leads to my missing some elements that I omit to hear or see, which restricts my understanding of the events and the process. As soon as I put myself into the protagonists' positions, ideas emerge as to which basic assumptions may have directed them. This means that the protagonists' material is interspersed with my associations, phantasms and assumptions, and retroactively I become a third in this process.

The first basic assumptions arise in the child's earliest psychic development through perceptual functions and early thought processes, and they smooth the child's path from inside to outside. These early sensory perceptions are condensed into images that can express pleasure and unpleasure. They are formed as crystallisation points of the early basic assumptions and they play a part in elaborating representations.

Early representations and early basic assumptions undergo reformulations by the subject in later life through experience and also through the subject's phantasmatic activity. Basic assumptions mature, unfold and develop in relationship to the object. In a transitional space, the external object is drawn into this play of the exchange, and the emerging dyad enables the subject's need (drive) for social interaction to nurture the exchange from inner to outer.

Representations and basic assumptions undergo maturation and allow the experience of time to develop. This suggests that there are different mature basic assumptions in the individual, so, there are also archaic basic assumptions that are fixed in perception. The more mature the basic assumptions, the more abstract they can become. Maturation also means that the subject can think about the basic assumptions and understand them in language.

Basic assumptions form part of the subject's behaviour. Archaic basic assumptions transformed by maturation form an ordered system that helps to regulate sensory input. I work from the assumption that in an individual's 'basic assumptions' system there are basic assumptions that conflict and clash and can turn against others.

Now what do these reflections specifically mean for my approach to this interview in image, sound and writing? I go through the interview and highlight the identifiable moments for me where the basic assumptions of Simone and/or the interviewer may be apparent. This was not about linking these moments more closely with the possible developmental history of Simone's respective basic assumptions that could be inferred from the prehistory and the boy's development. I try to follow the interview in such a way, I imagine, as to allow Simone's and the interviewer's basic assumptions to emerge in the interplay of the intersubjective relationship.

5.2.2 On the interview

I try to follow the interview according to how I conceive that Simone's and the interviewer's basic assumptions emerge in the interplay.

From the beginning up to the first drawing-play/squiggle:

Simone is 'on his guard'. He shows some mistrust at the beginning and makes clear his wish and desire to make contact with the object, the interviewer, as well as his fear of doing so, and in many ways indicates the following: 'the object wants something from me and I find that threatening. I don't know what it wants—but whatever it is, I'll reveal nothing and express the wish to look at the object through the mirror'.

Simone's supposed basic assumptions: 'I have no view through'; 'I need images'; 'the interviewer wants to confuse me'; 'I have only the representation of a *lacking*, living echo of the reliable object'; 'I only have available the representation of an unreliable object'. Connected with this are some further basic assumptions: 'I'm afraid of being discovered and at the same time feel the wish to be found'. 'The object is hidden, not reliable, uncertain and can mean danger. It unsettles me, wants to confuse me. The object could be intrusive'.

Simone now wants to show something of himself with pictures; he wants to draw. I read the interview—anticipating Simone's basic assumptions at this point—as if he were saying: 'I can't trust this object, on the one hand; on the other, I still dare in this space of "the transference" to align my ideas, feelings and phantasies with the real object'. 'I can't put difficult things into words; I only have images I can't translate into words. In this intermediate space, transitional space, I'm in danger of getting lost (lost in transition; lost in translation); when the images are captured in words, it gets worse. I have no secure internal language, no secure identity'.

The interviewer seems to work from the following basic assumptions: 'There is on the one hand a wish in Simone to confuse me and on the other hand an unconscious striving by him to enter into an interaction with me'. 'In these projective mechanisms of Simone's, I make myself available as a "malleable object", i.e. I allow myself to be confused'.

Simone emphasises the wish to be in a different place. Inside and outside are used in a confusing way. He would like not to be confused and not to be excluded but to be fusionally together with the object, as later portrayed in his drawings and in the playing. Simone is afraid of getting confused, in the way that he has probably already experienced elsewhere. 'There are things I'm ashamed of today (e.g. 'doing something stupid'). I want to turn things around (inside, outside), am confused and can also be confusing (shift from passive to active)'. 'I don't know how to make contact with the counterpart, because I don't know who the real object is, I don't have enough secure object-representations for that'. Simone emphasises this with: 'People keep not answering me'.

I think the interviewer assumes that Simone wants to be given attention and is at the same time afraid of it. Simone wants contact with the object but from a 'secure position'. He wants to 'know' and be there but at the same time to be 'invisible' (magic cloak) and 'secret'. Simone reiterates the urge and the wish for a relationship to the object and at the same time indicates fear of it. At this moment what is important is a clear space/framework that the interviewer shows Simone, which makes the contact easier. Simone's first contact in the transference with the interviewer consists in a defence by means of projective identification. Interviewer: 'I'm not the confusing object that Simone believes me to be'. Simone projects his confusion on to the interviewer; he doesn't want to be recognised. The interviewer can continue to function, although strong confusion impulses are proceeding from the patient; interviewer: 'I can mend myself. I can allow myself to be deformed and put myself back together'.

A person's structure can be homogeneous or heterogeneous. Simone's identity is not homogeneously constructed; it consists in partial structures. In different states, various core identities appear, connected with different representations. Simone does not always have access to all object-representations.

In this situation the interviewer suggests a 'solution': the squiggle game.

5.2.3 Squiggles

First squiggle: the interviewer prepares a way for Simone with a squiggle game. Simone shows that he does not understand this game; squiggling confuses him. Simone: 'I need a recognisable thing, an object, an image. I can do "something much better than a squiggle"'. Simone is again projecting confusion onto the interviewer, who seems to have the impression that the 'food' he is giving Simone is being rejected and is not good. When he makes or omits an intervention, an interpretation, it is in order to foster the psychoanalytic process.

Simone goes back to drawing and: 'I have the possibility of being able to create an object that is good for me, but I don't know how I should start on it, for when I try to create an object there is a crash. The crash and noise with the sirens bring about help by the activation of emergency mechanisms (KPA-vehicle). Then an emergency man (interviewer) appears, who can become experienceable for me. I'm carrying many burdens inside me and I've been hurt in an accident'.

The proximity now felt by Simone to the phantasmatic-destructive (crash) becomes intolerable for him. The interviewer cannot avoid withstanding Simone's paranoid fear. This holding enables the subject to develop a narrative. That appears to be possible for Simone only with regard to the object, i.e. in its presence. By the portrayal in the squiggle, early traumas are awakened in Simone. Simone: 'With narratives I can escape from dangerous situations'.

Second squiggle: the proximity to the destructive (crash) now felt by Simone is experienced by him as intolerable. It follows from this that he would like to do 'something big', a big squiggle that blocks the view of what is intolerable. He wants to create the picture entirely on his own. Water, waves with a mother-fish and a child-fish, appear—but then it quickly becomes disturbing again, threatening: a storm is brewing, from 'inside'; Simone: 'I can't tame the destructive, the threatening by changing the theme. Inside me is a hurricane that is churning up high waves. I feel violent affects inside me, drive impulses that I can't evade. I reject the interviewer's interpretation about the difficult, stormy time with mother, I can't tolerate it'. The hurricane and the waves are something that concern Simone himself, his object representations and also the current real-object. Simone makes some attempts at avoidance, by calming the waves. Yet then a new danger of devouring destruction threatens: the pelican (mother-representation? Father-representation?) appears in the story. The displacement on to the third is unconsciously an attempt fleetingly to eliminate the tension in the field between the fish and their environment. But the third is also dangerous. It should be destroyed but destruction is also frightening, as it could also affect Simone. 'I'm sparing no effort to escape destruction. To escape the danger of destruction (threatening collapse), I must plunge deep with the object, fusionally into the unconscious or rather into the depressive. Afterwards I must surface again but there I experience a depressive mood and confusion. Any move I make to escape destruction is accompanied by a regression in the object relationships (self-object)'. Extremely violent inner movements cannot be resolved externally either. What is threatening is everywhere; it leads to 'fight' and 'flight'. Simone now clearly shows that he needs some help.

It seems to me that the emerging transitional space eases the development of the transference (I think this is also the case for the interviewer), which allows Simone to feel some hope, for he shows some early approaches to using the interviewer as an object. Simone: 'Actually I'm not managing to calm inner storms. For this I'm reliant on help from the real object'. Simone now increasingly finds the session to be an experience with a 'good' object that can and should 'follow' him, which stirs in him a desire to experience more things with the 'interviewer' good object. 'I can attach the object to me with dangerous and funny stories, but I'm afraid the object will move away if it is no longer so funny and dangerous'. Then there is obviously a danger of threatening object loss and deprivation.

Third squiggle: Simone would like to have more time with the interviewer. It seems he has the idea that the time can be extended with stories. The interviewer draws a fox that is quickly recognised by Simone. Simone explains that the fox needs protection in a hole and wants to find some treasure. I understand 'treasure' ['Schatz'] as 'protection' ['Schutz']. Simone (the fox) cannot reach the treasure because there is a border there. The dangerous third, the pelican-father, can reach the treasure-mother (oedipal) but not the little fox-Simone. For the interviewer it is also a matter of withstanding Simone's paranoid fear.

In the drawings, a dangerous shark with lots of teeth, rows of teeth, now surfaces. In this session, Simone *together with* the interviewer imagines a shark. For the first time there is a 'we'. Simone's aggressive components emerge (teeth that grow back). These aggressive/defensive tools are omnipotently multiplied. Simone recoils from his own aggressiveness after discovering that he does not have just one dentition. A plaster with a skull has been placed over a wound on the shark-mother's belly. I wonder whether this is the wound after the birth of a child? The plaster is to let something heal up, but it simultaneously indicates the injury. Possibly there exists with a secure object in Simone a phantasy of being born again, being able to start again from the beginning.

Now the interviewer mentions the fact that two harmless fish can become dangerous predator fish. As I hear this, the interviewer is conveying there that what is threatening cannot be eliminated in that way. In other words: the aggressive shark, Simone's dangerous component, remains persistently threatening, but Simone repeatedly escapes the threat. Magical changes are easier for Simone to achieve than working through conflicts with a real object followed by new integration. Change is only possible in dialogical exchange with a real object.

Fourth squiggle: now there are some further changes. The small child-fish-Simone grows up and wants to have children—as a swordfish! The primal scene phantasy is not elaborated at all though. Nevertheless, for Simone this is about change. Simone would like change as transmutation … repeatedly: dangerous Simone-shark-components are to be transmuted, for transmutation is easier than integration and transformation. But Simone has an intuition: development and procreation only go together with an object.

The interviewer can restore his function that is being disturbed, distorted, impaired by the patient's transference. In the transference, the real object can be aligned with the phantasm. Then transformation is possible for Simone.

Fifth squiggle: the transmutation continues: mother-shark and child-shark are now hammerhead sharks that keep changing form. Transformation for Simone means becoming 'nicer' (more lovable). The magical-phantasmatic transmutation allows some calming and aids self-regulation.

Simone makes a potential new discovery: 'I can only develop a new representation of the real object if this is different from my previous object-representations'. At the end of the session, Simone does not want to hand over the stories, the session, the experience, but to keep them (take away the drawings).

5.2.4 Playing with the toy animals

The interviewer takes on the role of a dangerous animal that wants to eat. In the play Simone develops an 'as-if' anxiety because of the supposed threat from the interviewer. Simone wants to calm him down and feeds him some acorns. Then the theme of eating and being eaten develops further, and Simone begins to feel a mild anxiety that dangerous, aggressive components could also proceed from Simone and about how these would be dealt with. So he keeps transforming himself into other animals: squirrel, skunk.

For the interviewer this is a matter of allowing the distortion of the real object by Simone in the transference and overturning it by reconstruction and interpretation. He must become the 'bad' object and show that he is also a 'good' object. Simone now likewise considers a transformation from bad to good to be possible. So, Simone can use the object and strive for transformation or further development. But he recognises that it entails some psychic work to allow oneself to enter an object relationship. Nevertheless, he still has an intuition that further development is possible. In this context the fantasy can arise: I, Simone, can also be biblical, holy, spiritual, strong, invisible and carry the cross (for an object/for himself?). A magical solution opens up: I can develop myself further, then the 'bad components' that make it so difficult for me and are so confusing will disappear and then I will become a spiritual, an invisible Simone. It remains unclear whether this is about imitation or an identification.

In the play with the animals, the interviewer offers the possibility that the third person does not have to be only threatening, only excluded, only unpleasurable—since this would amount to a simplistic reduction of their characteristics and feelings—but that many more degrees of freedom and pleasurable possibilities are to be attributed to him.

5.2.5 Concluding remarks

In this interview Simone managed by means of the presence of the real object to look out a little at the interviewer from under the magic cloak and attempt some first integrations (to bring everything under one hat). Simone's neediness and wish for a development-fostering object clearly emerges. 'As reassurance and a guarantee that I have really had this experience, I would like to take the nice squirrel away with me'. The emergency number becomes important and, together with the ambulance (KPA) at the beginning of the drawings, forms a kind of framework for the encounter.

5.3 Commentary 3 (Kerstin Westhoff)

5.3.1 Introductory remarks

Engaging with various theoretical standpoints in psychoanalysis, discussions with colleagues in the context of my psychoanalytic training, the daily clinical work and, of course, my own analysis and supervisions have influenced my ways of thinking and working. The question as to my identity as a psychotherapist who takes a psychoanalytic approach and my 'professional self' is posed for me in a long-term continuing process of debate between basic theoretical standpoints and a living clinical reality.

Meticulous interrogation of my own basic assumptions with the aid of the clinical material made available to us here was a great challenge. On the one hand, there is the dimension of developed and considered basic assumptions that constitute the psychoanalyst's own identity, of which I am aware in my analytic-therapeutic attitude. On the other hand, there are complex, sometimes confusing situations with each counterpart in a highly specific therapeutic situation and my own psychic reality, but also rapid changes in present-day living realities that can flow into interventions and represent authentic working and situational, flexible reacting. The complex mixture of implicit and explicit basic assumptions leads to my own psychoanalytic way of working, which can be placed on a possible spectrum of other psychoanalytic ways of working, and I would like to bring out some of its aspects. However, just as my interpretations, associations and interventions initially only find paths into language through considerable detours, I have encountered some substantial difficulties. At first the work in the group led me to reconsider more precisely what the capacity to think analytically comprises for me personally but also the extent to which changed living realities in our contemporary present also represent new and different challenges for psychoanalysis. Psychoanalysis does not mean for me a convenient method that is available for me to use for all time. I do not see it as the source of a deep, obscure knowledge that I only need to tap appropriately to approach the treasures of knowledge. As Sandler wrote:

> To try to satisfy all "*explanatory intents*" with one comprehensive theory is clearly impossible, and I would urge the view that we have a *body of ideas*, rather than a consistent whole, that constitutes psychoanalytic theory. What is critical is not what psychoanalytic theory *should* be, but what should be *emphasised* within the whole compass of psychoanalytic thinking.
>
> (1983, p. 37, my italics)

Thinking and emotions tend to favour detours and byways, and insights often surprise us in inconspicuous places. For me working analytically means a thinking that moves forward associatively, does not allow itself to be deterred by impassable terrain, does not turn in on itself and retains for itself something refreshingly free-floating. But on which elements does the specific analytic dialogue now feed and how accessible are they to us? The psychoanalytic basic assumption that most of what concerns the mind is not consciously accessible gives rise to the task of finding a specific balance in the analytic dialogue: alternating between conscious and unconscious processes without an overemphasis on one or the other. Thoughts and associations do not arise at random. In the oscillating polar tension-field of complex analytic relational events with their specific setting, there arises against the background of my technical knowledge, my person, my associating, focusing, speech or silence a particular space of listening and attention that opens up both inwards and outwards. Interpretations and associations therefore appear to me most likely to be verbally conveyed messages that evoke my own images and are recaptured in language from my own unconscious and the analysand's unconscious, which I often do not manage to hear or perceive. But when and how do I reach the decision to speak or to be silent? Here I assume at a specific moment in the context of the analytic dialogue that my thoughts are appropriate to the other. The context of an analytic dialogue, in contrast to random interpersonal social encounters, is explicit and is specified by us. We thereby work from the basic assumption that it provides protection, mobilises the analysand's unconscious wishes and that a psychoanalytic process is set in motion by the context. According to that, the analytic setting would ease the transference and be especially well-suited to activating, observing and reflecting on the different movement forms of the transferences and countertransferences. Green has written that the setting should be constituted so as to create 'a ventilated space' that is 'neither the empty one nor one filled to overflowing' (1975, p. 8), so a space of possibility that creates as much presence and absence as is necessary for the formation of representations, for the representation of the object forms in its absence (Bion). With our associations and interventions, we contribute to preserving the 'ventilated' space. Designations create space and allow movement in the analytic dialogue. But when and why do we offer which setting?

Now in the following text I work from the above-mentioned basic assumption that certainties and securities do not blend with psychoanalytic thinking. Psychoanalysis therefore consists I think in an incessant questioning that always brings us closer to what is unsayable and inaccessible, and it challenges assumed knowledge and an exaltation of technique. Openness in analytic thinking should of course not be understood as the idealisation of not-knowing but as a constant critical reflection on deceptive certainties.

In what follows I will, with the aid of selected sequences, address the movements within the session as an entire procedure and assume with this way of proceeding that early forms of experiences are incorporated in a narrative context. Splinters and transferred elements will remain because every further engagement with the clinical material brings out new associations, new aspects and new perspectives, and this is why I understand my text as a kind of workshop-report.

5.3.2 *Progress of the sessions*

The session begins for Simone with a confrontation with the setting conditions under which the encounter with the analyst is taking place. The setting stipulates an asymmetry: you speak—I listen; you have your place—I have my place. The setting conditions of the protagonists in an analytic dialogue are probably always different at the beginning. The one-way mirror situation, the feeling of being subjected to the looks of others, the seated position assigned, the pre-defined timespan—all that seems to unsettle Simone very much at first, to arouse fears, extending to a sense of the uncanny. Having taken his place in the 'wrong' armchair, Simone is no longer in a position to give it away. Here transference is already in play: how will I (Simone) feel in the other's presence? What will he (the interviewer) say, what will I say? What kind of person is he? The setting, with its signs of beginning and ending, with its limitations, obviously seems threatening for Simone at first, like something that might dissolve his boundaries, so it is not a third in the positive sense but instead indicates a frightening third.

The interviewer now lets Simone explore and investigate the strange space and something meaningful happens. In this way he helps Simone to feel and find meaning through a shared experience. Simone's obvious discomfort is answered with this and perhaps even shared. The strong affects are picked up by the interviewer. What Simone felt obviously took precedence for the analyst at this point over why it was felt. Already here, at this early point in the interaction, the interviewer becomes a meaningful other, with whom perhaps also internal spaces can be explored and feelings can be mentioned, and there is the attempt at a first interpretation:

Interviewer: Are you a good observer?
Simone: Mm … Yes!
Interviewer: Yes? Have you got used to observing people? And would you actually like to be there, but so that you can't be seen? Like under a magic cloak?
Simone: Mm.

However, Simone still seems too excited actually to be able to receive an interpretation on this level (namely the expansion of meanings) at this point. If we assume that the precondition for explanatory interventions is a certain capacity to tolerate fear and pain and to endure thinking, we could put forward the hypothesis that this was not yet possible at the beginning of the session. At first the interviewer seems to understand Simone's behaviour—not wanting to show himself (the magic cloak)—as Simone's <u>attitude</u>.

Interviewer: ... And are people not to see you because they shouldn't know you want to know something?
At the moment that the interviewer receives Simone's unsettled state as behaviour that makes sense and has adaptive value, the relationship begins, and attachment begins to blossom.
Interviewer: ... But that could mean you're actually very afraid someone might discover you.

At this point Simone is in a position to formulate a first wish to the analyst: 'To know who <u>you</u> are!'

The first sequence leads me to think that there is probably a horizon of expectation for Simone that encompasses the fear of getting into a situation of alienation with the feeling of exposure and a lack of relationship on the one hand, and hope and the wish to feel answered and secure, on the other. At first, Simone seems to experience the setting specified here not as protection but as a 'reference function' in the sense of a worrying, confusing boundary. So he suddenly seems to find himself back in a situation that mobilises feelings of helplessness, uncertainty and powerlessness. Does Simone feel a radical difference here, a 'minus', a lack, connected with his person in contrast to the interviewer (to the 'overpowering' other)? The bi-personal space, the place of creativity, play and what is new, has not yet arisen. Simone confuses the interviewer, sends him into the void (*'Tee-hee!'*) and it takes a while for them to find a beginning.

The offering of alternative meanings (e.g. the *magic cloak* or: *'you're saying I'm just as you think I am'* or: *'something in you that sometimes confuses you?'* and *'afraid someone might discover you'* etc.) seems for Simone to indicate that painful difference where he may well experience the interviewer as too forcefully eloquent and overpowering.

Interviewer: There's nothing in you that confuses you
Simone: Yes there is.
Interviewer: What?
Simone: When people keep not answering me.

How therefore would Simone like to be answered? In an analytic encounter both partners in the dialogue take a certain risk, by uttering words with an almost endless meaning that can be charged with great intensity. It is the exploration of a potential abyss that separates two people and simultaneously the treading of a bridge that connects the two together. To be answered and recognised (coming out from under the magic cloak) is a great risk though for Simone, and so it is initially about trust and the question of what the interviewer wants from him. For the interviewer here, as in every initial interview or every session of an analytic dialogue, there is the potential risk of failing in the danger of not making contact and sticking exclusively to what is manifest.

Simone: Mm … isn't it just that you want to confuse me a bit, so that I say more?
Interviewer: I'm happy for you to tell me more, but I don't want to confuse you.
Simone: Yes you do.
Interviewer: I do?
Simone: Yes!
Interviewer: … and you don't believe what I'm telling you at all?
Simone: No, not at all!

Simone now tries to create a certain 'balance' in the squiggle game. He would like to show something, namely that he can already draw much better, '*something much better than a squiggle*'. Perhaps we might say with Simone: I certainly have no control over you, interviewer; you're not a part of me. But, by determining what I draw, I turn a passive experience into an active one. In this way, Simone learns something about himself but also about the other. He discovers that the combination of an initially threatening third (the setting) can go hand in hand with experiencing the interaction with a third person (the interviewer–father) with *recognition*. The interviewer's words therefore seem to Simone to allow the recognition of difference.

Interviewer: but that's a great story you've told me there, a very important one. I think that's a very exciting story you've made there, Simone, really!

It is not a subordination experienced as powerless and humiliating (which may have been one of Simone's basic assumptions) that happens here; instead a new experience becomes possible, which enables Simone to see himself from the other's perspective—not loaded with paranoid anxieties and fear. Simone now seems to be able to tolerate the difference much better and to enjoy a (sometimes silent) togetherness, without having to feel 'unanswered' and unconsidered or instead fused and so also non-existent.

Now the precondition for an emotional dialogue is there, allowing enough movement and scope and differences beyond the categories of good/bad, powerful/powerless, better/worse recognised.

Simone: I have ... that's a biblical name, 'Simone'.
Interviewer: That's right, what else do you know then about Simone, the
   biblical one?
Simone: Hm, ah yes, I, Simone carried the cross of Jesus up to the hill.

Language is a vehicle; it captures a feeling in a word and all these words
are connected with emotions—exhilarating, burdensome, frightening.
'Sentiment, intuition, intellectual or psychological illumination', writes
George Steiner, 'crowd at the inner edge of language, but cannot "break
through" to complete articulation' (2005, p. 19). It may be a basic assumption of Simone's that words are potentially dangerous, carry a burden that is
too heavy, too great, too threatening for him. Towards the end of the session,
the following scene takes place:

Simone: I'd like to play a game that goes quickly.
Interviewer: I don't know anything that goes quickly. Couldn't we just talk
   a bit more?
Simone: Hm *(indicating no)*. I've got another idea. There's a shark there
   isn't there? We could play with it a bit.

The analyst's fairly receptive attitude enables Simone to experience periods of
silence or moments in which the analyst is making notes not as a break in communication but as a 'space of possibility'. Simone dares more and more to open
up, to appear and to make contact with the interviewer. He does not have to feel
pressurised and '*always unanswered*'. Simone is in a position to outline and
build a complex, coherent phantasy sequence. He can now use his drawings and
his language for exchanging thoughts and making use of the interviewer. He
can reach Simone with simple, empathic or explanatory comments, both intel-
lectually and emotionally. I mean empathy here not in the sense of a capacity to
move from one world into another but to find the shared world.

After the beginning of the session when an uncertain and tense mood
prevailed, at the end of the encounter Simone can play together with the
analyst: pleasurably and combatively pressing ahead, eager–devouring,
fearful–flinching and also tender. Simone has a strong narrative skill, which
at the beginning of the session is still used entirely in the defence of helplessness but can then develop increasingly freely. At the end of the session, the hope for a dialogue with a meaningful other is movingly expressed
when Simone says: 'I like you' and a bit later: 'Shall we be friends?'

Simone can now dare to allow all these strong feelings and wishes. He
receives them for the moment and in the interviewer's presence '*under one
hat*'. Ambivalence can be tolerated (the squirrel develops further into the
skunk), renunciation is achieved and it is possible to say goodbye.

5.3.3 Afterthoughts

It is impossible to speak about everything. Not everything can be reported, either about a concluded analysis or about the course of a session. It is impossible to think about everything and to follow every association. In engaging with the present clinical material, I made a selection and discovered in the process that an emotionally supported (subjective) feeling of coherence about the 'reality' of Simone's psychic processes has started in me and I had serious difficulties in putting back in question a thought once it was thought, or an association. By coherence I do not of course mean in this context that it is coherent in the sense of being a 'truth'. In any case the engagement with the basic assumption of openness and tolerance towards not-knowing and not-understanding that is important to me led me to enquire again as to what may be impeding or fostering my free attitude in analyses and how much work the basic assumption that certainties and securities do not blend with psychoanalytic thinking actually demands of us. This would be in Winnicott's sense the place where creativity and play arise.

5.4 Commentary 4 (Angelika Staehle)

5.4.1 Explicit basic assumptions of the psychoanalytic situation

I work from the assumption that in the psychoanalytic setting—in a bipolar field—between the patient and the analyst, the patient portrays elements of his inner world. Both psychoanalyst and patient are actors in a common scene with an unconscious meaning that becomes representable through the preconscious and can then be grasped in language and so become accessible to consciousness. How the internalised relational-representations are externalised depends though on ego-maturity and on whether these are representations that are symbolised or experiences that were excluded from further psychic development by early inadequate holding/containment by primary objects encysted in the psyche. These are not communicable through words but appear in actions (rhythm, speed) and through the body like gestures, facial expressions, sense impressions and excitations. They can often only be inferred from the atmosphere in a session.

I try in the session with the patient not only to take up what he communicates to me with words but also to make myself available as a sounding board with all my senses and my body. In my interventions I try to capture descriptively in words what I hear, see and sense. I understand the analytic setting as a space that allows the patient to use the analyst increasingly and a shared third to arise with him. The quality and the function of the third can then be examined and processed. The space with two isolated individuals becomes an intermediate space shared by both. That means a space that is dominated by no one, in which each has space for what is his own—with reference to Green's 'well-ventilated space', a space that allows some air to breathe.

Which fundamental basic assumptions underpin my understanding of the psychoanalytic situation? From the outset of life, the human being needs an other in order to become a subject that can understand himself and others in a comprehensive way. We must first be understood before we can understand others. This contains the assumption that there is an innate expectation that there will be an other who takes up my physical and psychic needs and responds to them. There is from the outset of life in every baby a quest to be recognised and answered. I, as the other, assume that I can connect, understand and convey to him something of the other person's offered conscious and unconscious elements. Through the gradual internalisation of these functions, development and psychic change become possible.

5.4.2 Implicit basic assumptions

I do not have unconscious, implicit basic assumptions directly accessible to me that are rooted in my internalised relational representations and their accompanying affects and forms of defence. The context of my professional training and my integration in institutional structures also have an impact. To maintain access to all this I need others, as for example in the supervision or intervision.

5.4.3 My listening and my perspective on the interview with Simone

My basic assumptions, both explicit and implicit, determine how I hear both Simone's and the interviewer's basic assumptions. I try to infer Simone's basic assumptions and those of the interviewing psychoanalyst from the interview (transcript and video) made available to us. In the initial scene, when the way of proceeding with the one-way mirror is being explained, I think Simone's and the interviewer's different basic assumptions are portrayed as follows:

Simone has no confidence in an object that can understand him. He does not want to come out and be observed. 'I'd be happy if I were in there' (in the room behind the one-way mirror). Simone overplays his anxiety by trying to be the actor, i.e. to be the one who is observing. He strives to move on to the level of action: 'Why don't we do it the other way round: they [the group observing behind the one-way mirror] can sit here, and we'll sit over there?'

The interviewer has confidence though that he can get to know Simone and understand him. He picks up Simone's form of defence, his fear of the object's gaze; he finds a metaphor for it ('magic cloak') and suspects that Simone's need to know something is to remain unacknowledged.

As I heard the scene, Simone is also looking for a demarcating and protective envelope—in a completely bodily way: '*I'd be happy if I were in there*' (he is referring to the small side-room). There Simone would be protected from paranoid fears because he has not, so I suppose, internalised a protective 'psychic skin'. Therefore, he needs a magic cloak as a replacement skin, which however hinders his further development. He can only be curious and emerge when he feels safer. Emerging is dangerous. Here an externalisation of one of Simone's object representations already appears, which is confusing and contradictory, which he cannot trust. I sense Simone's need very acutely.

The interviewer can withstand Simone experiencing him as someone who wants to confuse him. Simone expects not to be understood but to be confused and protects himself against this by confusing others.

The interviewer persists: he would like them both to get to know each other. Simone is lacking the connection between feelings and words. He would like to draw something but also to show something of himself, but he cannot communicate it in words. 'I've done something stupid', says Simone, about why he has come.

When the interviewer continues trying to find out what Simone means by this, the object representation appears: '*Mm, isn't it just that you want to confuse me a bit, so that I say more?*'

The interviewer explores further how Simone experiences him. His basic assumption that it is an important step to make Simone's projective identifications accessible to him becomes apparent: '*But, you know, perhaps there's something in you that sometimes confuses you?*'

Simone's basic assumption, it seems to me, is as follows: how can I test whether the interviewer is helpful or threatening as an object? To the interviewer's question: '*There's nothing in you that confuses you?*' Simone explains, '*When people keep not answering me*'.

I hear this sentence as something that I connect with traces of Simone's life history: having received confusing messages from the primary object mother, having been confronted with an object that had not 'answered' him adequately. By that I mean a mother who had not been able to 'hold' the child's archaic emotional expressions, deal with them appropriately or respond to them verbally but projected her own unprocessed feelings onto the baby and later onto the child.

The interviewer sticks with the line that Simone wants to confuse him and to stay under the magic cloak because he has a terrible fear of being discovered. Yet Simone keeps to his basic assumption that he must first test the object: 'To know who you are!'

5.4.4 Squiggles

5.4.4.1 First squiggle

The interviewer takes up Simone's wish to draw and suggests a squiggle game. His basic assumption seems to be that Simone can accept the game of creating something together.

Simone's basic assumption may be: then I'll be drawn into something, I'll be destroyed. In the transitional space, the demarcation is no longer secured for Simone. 'Mixed proportions' unsettle him, it seems to me. Simone: 'I don't understand what you mean' (he shakes his head). He takes up the rhythm in his squiggle, but the two squiggles remain separate.

Simone now draws a car with a mop-head antenna and horn. At the front is a lorry with KPA written on it, as Simone says. He is now the only actor with <u>his</u> drawing—he feels safe with a drawing that originates from him alone. Protected in this way from a confusion by the other, he can use the object, i.e. form a new object representation. There is an antenna, a horn and then the emergency man. Later in the conversation it becomes clear: there was an accident on the motorway with a child from the children's psychiatric department (KPA). The interviewer asks: 'And help is urgently needed?' to which Simone says: 'Yes!'

The interviewer in this section of the interview is a counterpart, a real object, who poses enlightening questions. By drawing and aided by the object's presence, Simone can show something of himself. Yet his story must remain in the picture. Simone cannot yet take up a reference back to him made in language (the interviewer asks 'Do you think it could be that Simone is actually telling me he may urgently need help?'). Yet, after enquiring, he can moderate the urgency and say: 'I think so too'. Here a movement appears to a less threatening object representation, which enables him to make more use of the object.

5.4.4.2 Second squiggle

Now Simone can let himself get involved as the interviewer makes a squiggle and he joins in. Simone sees 'water' in the interviewer's squiggle. He paints waves and then a big mother-fish and another big fish, both are in a stormy sea, caused by a hurricane. As he amplifies elements of the drawing, Simone can with the help of the interviewer's empathetic, constantly questioning accompaniment, create fragments out of his history with his mother. A basic assumption of Simone, namely that there could be support from a present father, surfaces now in the form of some hope. An intervention by the interviewer, commenting that the drawing might be a portrayal of his history with his Mum, he can only half-accept on being asked.

The pelican introduced by Simone would like to catch the fish. Simone declares: '*Yes, now something dangerous is coming with the pelican*'. The pelican becomes the thief. I wonder: is the father the third, the dangerous one, or/and are these Simone's own aggressive drive excitations? But there is also 'a man ... he's carrying a gun because he's protecting the fish'. Here a basic assumption of Simone's surfaces, that aggression could also serve as protection. Yet, because of the successive transmutations, this seems really precarious.

The interviewer picks up that the danger surfaces in various transmutations; at first it was dangerous for the fish and now it is for the pelican. Next Simone draws a wall into which the pelican is banging its head. Yet the wall is partly permeable: '[the fish] can get to the other side of the sea; the fish don't have to experience the threatening danger; they can get through there. But they have to go a long way down ... and then a long way up, as far as they have to go down'.

The man who protects with the gun has become a wall that only blocks—a father who does not stand firm, disappears or is threatening? Such a father figure, which provides no help for the conversion of aggression, makes Simone's own aggression seem threatening.

The fish can escape by diving deep down into another sea. For Simone that could mean he has no confidence that he can withstand a threat, defend himself appropriately and receive help but that he only gets away by withdrawing emotionally and tuning out the danger. The rescue is then by another sea—another mother? A possible basic assumption of Simone's could be: there is yet another mother-representation.

5.4.4.3 Third squiggle

Simone would like to make another story. He has become curious and suggests to the interviewer that he should also do something like that. Then the interviewer draws a fox, introducing something new. Simone partly identifies with the fox who needs a den. There is some treasure that the fox/Simone would like to have. Desire and wishes to steal appear. There is also a spade; the fox is given a mouth and eyes by Simone. Then Simone develops the picture of a shark with sharp teeth and even double teeth. My basic assumption that forms at this point is as follows: Simone's desire to dig out the treasure becomes dangerous.

The doubling of the rows of teeth indicates a basic assumption of Simone's, namely that it is dangerous to have teeth—to integrate the aggressive impulses as his own. A way out consists in having two rows of teeth at the same time, then there is no loss. If one row of teeth has gone, there is a replacement available. For Simone this is about the reduction of danger, it is about survival, not further development. The two little fish have turned into predator fish: 'on the way they ate a lot, then they became little predator fish!'

The interviewer talks about growing up and refers to the approaching change of teeth, i.e. to development. Then Simone draws a skull on the shark: 'One he's eaten, a bit, or it's still alive'. Another basic assumption of Simone's becomes clear: sharks are constantly also threatened themselves, yet somehow they get away. Living/non-living is reversible.

5.4.4.4 Fourth squiggle

Simone: *So*, there's the great big sea again, look now, another stone like that … the smaller [fish] has grown up and has had a little baby; do you know why? … Because the mother has died and that was the girl.

Simone wrestles with change. Yet the mother is dead and the father is a stone. How is it possible to develop there? Simone's basic assumption here seems to me to be that survival is only possible by magical, omnipotent transformation.

The interviewer makes connections by formulating a story from Simone's fragments: 'So here some time has passed on the land, the Mummy has died, and the little girl has become a big woman, that's now just a boy, but how did this baby come about?'

Simone: 'Those are now swordfish' that he confirms can have babies on their own. For Simone there is only one sex; male and female in one. His basic assumption could be: gender differences are dangerous, one must control everything and be everything at the same time. In contrast, the interviewer works from the basic assumption that a third emerges from two, a man and a woman.

5.4.4.5 Fifth squiggle

Simone draws two new sharks and would like to know from the interviewer whether he knows these fish. The hammerhead sharks are clearly recognisable. With this question, Simone dares to use the interviewer for the first time. The interviewer names them and notices that they are big dangerous fish that like to eat. His basic assumption seems to be that this is about Simone's aggressive drives and drive phantasies.

For Simone there is only transmutation: 'They keep turning into another fish, then another, and another, always another'. In my view this defence contains a basic assumption of Simone's: he has magical powers. When the interviewer relates the transmutation to Simone, 'how is it then with

Simone—can he also change form?', Simone replies: '*Yes, become nicer*'. It appears that Simone can only split off the 'being bad' and escape it through transmutation. The interviewer brings to expression both parts of Simone: 'there's a bad Simone somewhere, then also a nice Simone, and he changes form'. To this Simone replies: 'And some day even a religious Simone … I'm invisible'. By linking the various parts of Simone, the interviewer now triggers the appearance of the invisible Simone. This is a new image for the magic cloak, also an omnipotence phantasy that is more connected with Simone.

To the interviewer's question: 'how do you get the nice, the bad and all the other Simones together under one hat?', Simone can reply: 'I don't know yet either'. He is able to take up something here. In this scene Simone's and the interviewer's basic assumptions concur, namely that it must be confusing with Simone's three parts.

5.4.5 Continuation of the story with the toy animals in the room

The story begins with a squirrel and a crocodile. The interviewer says: 'So I'm the big crocodile and I'm hungry?' A game of eating and being eaten develops between the two protagonists. The squirrel-Simone becomes the skunk-Simone. Interviewer: 'Simone seems to be quite a complicated person'. Simone: 'that's a biblical name, Simone … Simone carried the cross of Jesus up to the hill'. Interviewer: 'Yes, so you're actually a very strong person?'

Simone would like to take the squirrel away with him, to which the interviewer says: 'you're hungry for the squirrel'. The interviewer alludes here to a drive-related, possessive hunger for the object. The transmutation that Simone always seeks as an expedient is now lived out by them both in an enjoyable play-fight. At the end of the session Simone can express hope: 'I like you … Shall we be friends?'

The interviewer summarises the playing: 'sometimes [Simone] doesn't know how he can bring together all the various "Simone parts" that are there next to each other' and 'Perhaps, Simone, that's a task for this time you're spending with us, for you to try to put all these parts together'.

The interviewer's basic assumption becomes clear that development only proceeds by an integration of split-off Simone-parts. Simone has experienced hunger for a father and has developed curiosity in the sense of wanting to get to know someone. Simone conveys his basic assumption that he needs a counterpart with whom he can learn to tolerate variety and that he can use this other person in that way for his development.

Simone has relaxed his defence in the course of the interview. He has discovered that drive-related and related playing is possible. Simone was increasingly able to use the interviewer in Winnicott's sense. At the end of the session, his hope is expressed that there is something living that he would like to preserve. To that extent it can be said that Simone was able to use the adult in the interview to make connections between various representations.

References

Bion W. R. (1962): *Learning from Experience*. London: Tavistock.

Bollas C. (2015): *When the Sun Bursts. The Enigma of Schizophrenia*. New Haven/London: Yale University Press.

Cycon R. (1994): Preface to Klein's collected works. *Gesammelte Werke*, I, 1.

Faimberg H. (2019): Faimberg's method: 'Listening to Listening'. Intercultural and intracultural discussion groups. In: *Contribution of IPA Working Parties to Clinical Research in Psychoanalysis*. In press.

Freud S. (1900): *The Interpretation of Dreams*. SE 4.

Freud S. (1901): *The Psychopathology of Everyday Life*. SE 6.

Freud S. (1908a): *Creative Writers and Day-Dreaming*. SE 9.

Freud S. (1908b): *Hysterical Phantasies and their Relation to Bisexuality*. SE 9.

Green A. (1975): The analyst, symbolization and absence in the analytic setting (On changes in analytic practice and analytic experience)—in memory of D. W. Winnicott. *Int. J. Psychoanalysis*, 56, 1–22.

Kentridge W. (2014): *Six Drawing Lessons*. Cambridge, MA: Harvard University Press.

Kentridge W. (2017): A defence of the less good idea. Sigmund Freud lecture (recording).

Kentridge W. (2019): That which I do not remember. In: Kentridge W. (2019): *A Poem that is Not Our Own*. Cologne: W. König. pp. 93–103. (recording in English).

Klein M. (1932): *The Relations between Obsessional Neurosis and the Early Stages of the Super-Ego*. London: Hogarth Press, International Psychoanalytic Library.

Klein M. (1936): Weaning. In: *Love, Guilt and Reparation and Other Works, 1921–1945. The Writings of Melanie Klein*, Vol. I. London: Hogarth Press.

Sandler J. (1983): Reflections on some relations between psychoanalytic concepts and psychoanalytic practice. *Int. J. Psychoanalysis*, 64: 35–45.

Steiner G. (2005): Ten (possible) reasons for the sadness of thought. *Salmagundi*, 146/147, Spring–Summer, 3–32.

Winnicott D. W. (1971): *Playing and Reality*. London: Tavistock.

Winnicott D. W. (1973): *Therapeutic Consultations in Child Psychiatry*. London, Hogarth, 1971.

Note

1 Kentridge (2017) has described similar processes in the artist.

6 Discussion and experiences from the group's working method

This is a matter of highlighting the specificity and differentness with which each analyst works, with the aid of basic assumptions that become identifiable. This brings to light not only what distinguishes each analyst from another, but also which parts of which schools in what way had been integrated into his 'style'. The notion that every person in concrete terms proceeds somewhat differently already implies a basic assumption, namely that the 'other' is different. Basic assumptions comprise on the one hand theoretical-clinical metapsychological concepts and on the other hand ideas about the dynamics and the interplay of unconscious and conscious processes. But they also contain, for example, conscious and preconscious notions about internal and external, about communicative processes and structures and about the selectivity of hearing and speaking or of inner perception, understanding, processing and admittance, as well as the separation between what is one's own and what is alien.

To every analyst a part of his own basic assumptions is known and conscious. Basic assumptions that have not yet become conscious can enter into an open discourse supported by trust from the obscure-preconscious into the brightness of intellectual understanding. A basic assumption about basic assumptions is that we become aware only in reflective processes of the diversely complex composition of our mosaic of basic assumptions that exists at a specific point in time and their flexible creation. This mosaic changes over the course of every analyst's life. If an analyst goes back through his earlier notes from a high-frequency treatment many years later, this will become completely obvious to him. We are no longer the people we were, and we are not yet the people we become. In the exchange about specific clinical 'material', we move—stimulated by our conversation partner—out of the position of not knowing and not understanding ourselves and the other into this one of partly and temporarily knowing and understanding a little of ourselves and the other. Babylon, i.e. confusion in the use of different concepts and different kinds of definitions of the same concepts,

DOI: 10.4324/9781003304340-6

is a universally known phenomenon. We are thus not only reliant in ourselves on a constant work of translation (for example to transfer preverbal processes into verbal ones) but also on how much of what we have said has been understood and how we understand the counterpart's communications. With the technique of 'listening to listening', Faimberg (2019) introduced a methodology that makes it possible to reveal basic assumptions in various situations, i.e. between individual people or in groups and to work out misunderstandings creatively.

A development-fostering dialogue in Spitz's (1983) sense occurs in a transitional domain (Winnicott). The result corresponds to a spontaneous and improvised co-creation by all participants. Here the contributions by each author do not blur into a homogenous mush but function as relays that motivate the counterpart to perceive his own possibilities in the play and the development of the dynamics, possibly all the better the more difficult the task. We translate communication offers from others and the others translate ours. Empathy is helpful here but in no way guarantees freedom from 'errors'. The capacity for anticipation sometimes allows an 'advance reading' of the messages from the counterpart or from the other. What happens fairly often, however, is a 'mis-reading' in the sense of a parapraxis—even with the most appropriate attention. The process of clarifying ambiguous communication processes, including their primary sources, reveals the participants' basic assumptions increasingly clearly. The common element then consists in the work of reflecting on the differentness of the vertices (Bion) and the respective harmonies of each participant's basic assumptions in this process.

An analyst's set of basic assumptions is differently activated in various situations. This may happen in a way not too dissimilar to how key biological processes are currently conceptualised. For example epigenetic influences—which can change under the influence of environmental factors—determine the expression of genetically present information. In other words, the genetic orchestration in the genome is constant, but when which instruments play together and how—like a changing score—is determined by epigenetically modified external world factors. By analogy we can imagine that in a similar way a different pattern of intrapsychic understanding is activated on the one hand by the patient and on the other hand by the discussion of the corresponding 'material' in a group (epigenetic factors).

The wish to be able to foresee the future, i.e. to have prophetic abilities, belongs to the armoury of infantile omnipotence. Our understanding is always retrospectively focused. We divide up what we hear according to categories of understanding that generate a fairly satisfying picture of events according to the basic assumptions contained in them. From some point seen in an anterograde way, by means of the projection of past events, only an outline of what is to come in the future can be formed. Without reflecting on our own basic assumptions in the present, there is a danger that in what is to come we only find the treasure that we ourselves have already buried in the past. Only disciplined acquiescence allows outlines for the future to emerge in our understanding of relational events and at the same time for these to be removed again in order not to block our way, so that we can follow cognitive, emotional and drive-related events that are partly shaped by other people.

With active interest and a respectful attitude that fully accepts the other viewpoint without taking it on oneself, the goal of a corresponding dialogue or polylogue does not consist in reaching the decision as to whether a viewpoint is right or wrong, but in being able to understand the basis for the difference. It is never one of the key basic assumptions to assume that everything is equally significant, nor that any way of proceeding would be appropriate and equally valuable. It is only by careful and considerate analysis that our own base-assumptions belonging to the core of the personality, thinking, feeling, conceptualising and dialoguing become clear. At that point the feeling arises of hardly being able to change one's own viewpoint any longer and having to apply a great deal of effort to feel any empathy towards the counterpart's perspective.

In a group, clinical material assumes a specific, individual shape and meaning for each participant. The view integrated by a functional working group about the communicative structure of the clinical 'material' can only arise there, or alternatively, where the group is dysfunctional, also be destroyed by a collective using suggestion.

Our group reached the conviction that it is impossible to think without basic assumptions, even if these are found to be changing, i.e. we cannot get rid of basic assumptions. There seem to be various levels of basic assumption. In psychoanalytic conceptualising, there is no space free of basic assumptions. Basic assumptions create a certain stability, but also a restriction. They can be developed and scrutinised. They change in the course of an interview, depending on the particular object-relationship and the quality of the dialogue. Changes occur specifically with shocks or deep dismay. It is likely that the flexibility and elasticity of the basic assumptions of people who are in dialogue together acquire great significance when this concerns the perception of differentness rather than partisan struggles, the work of persuasion or claims to exclusivity. For basic assumptions to be perceived and potentially also modified, what is needed in the setting of communicative events are interpersonal transitional realms that make clear what is one's own, what is the other's and finally also what is co-created.

The further back basic assumptions are traced, the greater the reliance on biological basic assumptions of the body ego, which with their fundamental psychosomatic and somatopsychic components supply the basic materials for archaic phantasms and are shaped specifically in the corresponding cultural context.

In our discussions, we encountered many questions that remain open, as we did not want to get enmeshed in belief systems. We entered frontier regions in which basic assumptions were only recognisable schematically or only as outlines, the cohesion of unities loosened and the territory of not-knowing expanded. Already just in the question as to whether the drives and the unconscious are biologically constituted or are imported in Laplanche's sense from outside into the subject, i.e. whether our psychic origin is in the other or in ourselves, or whether in a circular process both are true, we found it difficult to determine or construct an effective basic assumption to this effect in the preconscious.

We developed relatively similar attitudes on the question of whether transference is not in fact a general, unavoidable phenomenon of interpersonal communication, with which we can only work in the analytic situation because we use a framework that with its asymmetric division of tasks makes the transference movements visible and 'comprehensible'. Nevertheless, we were agreed that any answer has many technical implications for the beginning, development and conclusion of an analytic treatment and not least can also give indications as to when interpretations of the transference are helpful and necessary and when it seems more appropriate to make interventions in the transference. The repercussions of these considerations on the structures of our training institutions, which often generate discontent, may be considerable (Zwettler-Otte, 2019). This in particular is also because the working in our group was generally felt to be enjoyable.

We worked from a highly unified basic assumption, namely that the psychoanalytic process is useful for processes that the subject, with regard to his mental development, cannot carry out alone (transferences and not only transference phantasies are only possible with real others). It is part of the human condition that, especially in childhood, but still also later on, people need other people. For certain developmental steps, a counterpart is indispensable. If there are large and indissoluble discrepancies between the basic assumptions of those interacting, whether these are children and adults or patients and analysts, problems arise. If there is an excessive adaptation to the other's basic assumptions, the developing child forms, like the patient in the analytic process, a false self, pseudo-movements ensue and the analyst may be caught by a deception that everything is as already verbally formulated by theory. He enjoys the confirmation of his ready-made concepts and his therapeutic wishes and loses his investigative curiosity.

The basic assumptions of the first year of life are probably not formulated yet in language but find expression through processual sequences of action/behaviour. Perhaps at some later date a series of basic assumptions about development could be formulated.

Representations, i.e. memory units that are formed securely in connection with a particular object from birth onwards (this point in time seems to be a basic assumption) can hardly be characterised as basic assumptions but rather as archives of relational episodes that contain the accompanying affects and corresponding contexts. What psychic energy they have available to be activated and to supply the contents to the fantasy activity of the primary process, i.e. by what legitimacies the ego cathects them or withdraws the libidinous or aggressive cathexis from them, seems to us to be largely obscure. An analogy could be drawn between a set of genetically given representational images and Freud's postulated primal fantasies, which he termed 'phylogenetic endowment' (1917, p. 371). There could certainly therefore also be constitutional differences in relation to the capacity to develop fantasies, to symbolise or to be scenically creative. Actual representations initially form in meaningful, interpersonal communicative dialogue between adults and babies/children/adolescents, i.e. between hormonalised, sexualised adult beings and infantilely sexualised persons not yet exposed to higher doses of sexual hormones. How does a baby/child use an adult? What does the adult have to offer the baby/child in the dialogue?

If we consider a child as a being who interprets himself, symbolises, and translates interactions into relational unities as well as developing his own theories, he certainly shapes, probably based on both innate and interactively acquired factors, the effects of the adult environment in an active way. Nevertheless, the external forces at work are mostly, in comparison to the child's activity, too strong. So special attention must be given to the relationship between self-interpretation or stranger-interpretation and the way in which it changes.

The development of the communicative system and the storing in it seemed to us hypothetically to occur approximately in the following sequence: first, perceptions such as visual forms, sounds, smells or tactile experiences with the development of a primary symbolism, then—with an increasing capacity for figurability in the visual domain—the construction of images and image sequences that are formed into the first averbal thoughts, then verbal, secondary symbolism that uses words, sentences, sequences of thoughts, texts and scenes. The more sequence, the more multi-dimensional connections as well. Words thus begin to carry an ever more complex communicative-emotional burden. Are there also basic assumptions for storing objects, images, i.e. very generally, forms? Can Kant's a priori forms be regarded as basic assumptions? 'But whereas a sign signifies an object, form signifies only itself' (Focillon, 1942, p. 3).

The meaning of deferred action, i.e. the ongoing reworking and transformation of any memory according to the state of ego-development and the respective drive dynamics in these processes, cannot be overestimated. The reciprocal effect of retrospective and prospective fantasising and retroactive revision assumes great importance here.

Both protagonists bring their inner spaces into the analytic process (transitional spaces, anxiety spaces, empty spaces; finally, the counterpart's spaces internalised in the earliest relationships) and scenarios as a different third into the real dialogue space. Each of the two reacts unconsciously to the other's 'gift' and conveys with it a piece of his own attunement. Spaces have to do with the body and its openings or the experiences that the individual has had with them up to a specific point in time. There may be some innate knowledge (another possible basic assumption) concerning endo-corporeal spaces that are specifically shaped in interaction and development.

One of the analyst's basic assumptions may consist in the idea: I make all of myself available to the patient in the asymmetric relationship, so that change can arise: body, psychic attunement, openness, and I allow my personal preconscious to be moved. But I thereby lose my security, and this—in relation to the later psychophysical restitution of the analyst's autonomy—is extremely strenuous.

The 'search-system' described in mammals (Panksepp, 1998), a form of cerebral analogy for the drive concept, involves genetically given assumptions about what is or should be sought in the environment (e.g. food, the breast), since after all the young of a primate cannot exist as a solitary creature. These can be imagined as innate behavioural schemas. The infantile sexual, which leans on the connatal self-preservative impulses, may contain pre-defined aspects of pleasurably and unpleasurably orientated basic assumptions.

The drive (our conscious basic assumption) is a force proceeding entirely from the somatic, which is directed by the intrapsychic, bodily as a source into the outside world. It is necessary for life and survival. Drive wishes open up psychic processes; taboos and phobic attitudes close them. With the 'openings', as with 'closing' taboos, there are cross-generational transmissions.

It is possible that various intrapsychic processes are also geared towards integrative movements. How far do the drive impulses arising from the unconscious traumatise the ego when there is no good enough environment available to take over the direction and regulation in the interpersonal field in an appropriate way? Holding is necessary for a narrative coherence to develop. Magical change is easier to achieve than integration and real change. The last two transformations are only possible with the aid of a real object. A patient's material has a certain inner coherence that is unknown to either protagonist in the clinical process. It can be worked out in retrospect; in what is present it is often barely perceptible. Figuration, i.e. the tendency to assemble something diffuse into something figurative, formed, is a precondition for integration. Where is the unthought and unrepresented placed?

The psychoanalytic-psychotherapeutic working alliance is shaped both by the patient's and the therapist's basic assumptions. Those of the patient (and of the analyst) are manifested mainly in the capacity for construction and in the (counter-transference). They become apparent in their conscious and preconscious phantasies.

References

Faimberg H. (2019): Basic theoretical assumptions underpinning 'Faimberg's method 'Listening to listening'. *Int. J. Psychoanalysis*, 100/3, 447–426.

Focillon H. (1942): *The Life of Forms in Art*. Translated by Charles Beecher Hogan and George Kubler. New Haven, CT: Yale University Press.

Freud S. (1917): The paths to the formation of symptoms (Lecture 23). In *Introductory Lectures on Psycho-Analysis*. SE 16.

Panksepp J. (1998): *Affective Neuroscience. The Foundations of Human and Animal Emotions*. Oxford University Press.

Spitz R. (1983): *Dialogues from Infancy*. Ed. R. N. Emde. New York: Oxford University Press.

Zwettler-Otte S. (2019): *Das Unbehagen in psychoanalytischen Institutionen. Konflikte, Krisen und Entwicklungspotenziale in Ausbildung und Berufsausübung* [Discontent in psychoanalytic institutions. Conflicts, crises and development potential in training and professional conduct]. Gießen: Psychosozial-Verlag.

7 Summary

We are drawing on Bion in using the term 'basic assumptions'. These are explicit or implicit convictions that play a key part in the processes of understanding, evaluating, ordering, anticipating and monitoring. Analytic listening is partly shaped by the basic assumptions of both the analyst and the patient.

In a working group of four analysts over two years, a transcribed, video-recorded interview with a child was studied individually then discussed in the group, with respect to the group members' different base-assumptions. Their different ways of hearing and understanding the material were worked out and portrayed in the group discourse. Our group reached the insight that it is impossible to think without basic assumptions, even if these may be changing, i.e. that *basic assumptions cannot be removed*. In psychoanalytic conceptualising, there is no space that remains free of basic assumptions. Basic assumptions create a certain *stability*, but also *restriction*. They can be *developed* and *questioned*. They *change* in the course of an interview, according to the respective object relationship and the quality of the dialogue. We thereby had the experience of how helpful and enjoyable the reciprocity turned out to be in the disclosure of each individual's own basic assumptions. The associated connection with many existing concepts and theories (e.g. unconscious phantasies) was also very stimulating.

DOI: 10.4324/9781003304340-7

Index

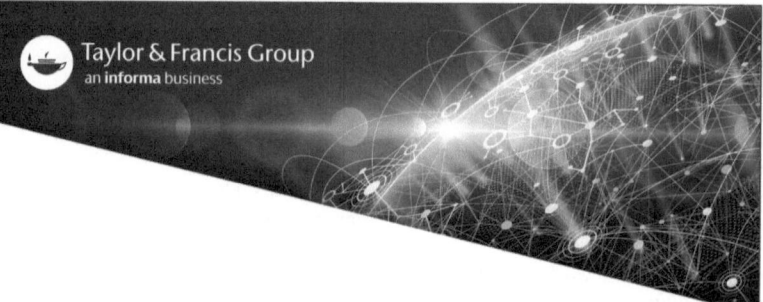
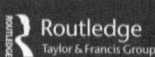
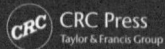

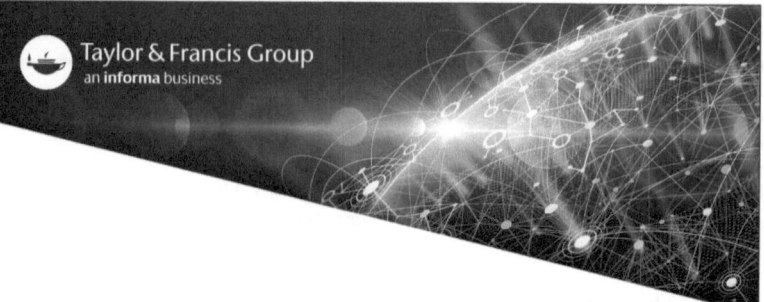
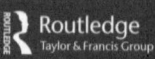
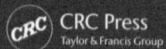